Author's Note

Thank you for picking up *The Green Elixir: Unlocking the Health Benefits of Nature's Most Powerful Plants.* As you explore the pages of this book, I hope you feel as inspired as I did while writing it. My journey into the world of plant-based wellness started with a simple curiosity about nature's incredible healing potential. What began as a personal exploration into healthier living soon grew into a deep admiration for the plants that have been used for centuries to nurture and restore the body.

I'm not a trained expert or a health professional, but rather an enthusiastic learner, eager to share the knowledge I've gathered along the way. In today's fast-paced world, it's easy to forget how much wisdom we can draw from the natural world around us. This book is my humble attempt to reconnect us with that ancient knowledge, offering practical and accessible ways to harness the power of plants in our daily lives.

Every plant in these chapters holds a special place in my heart. As you read about their healing properties, I encourage you to see them not just as remedies, but as gifts from nature. Each one has its own story to tell, and by incorporating them into our lives, we're not just improving our health, but also honoring the traditions that have valued them for generations.

This book isn't just about learning new facts; it's about starting a new way of thinking and living. It's about exploring how we can integrate the power of plants into our routines, using nature's wisdom to support our overall well-being. Whether you're a seasoned wellness advocate or someone just beginning to explore the benefits of plant-based living, I hope this book serves as a helpful guide on your journey.

Thank you again for joining me on this adventure. May you find inspiration, healing, and a deeper connection to the natural world as you unlock the green elixirs that nature has so graciously provided.

With gratitude,

Caterinah Muiruri.

The Green Elixir: Unlocking the Health Benefits of

Nature's Most Powerful Plants

The Green Elixir: Unlocking the Health Benefits of
Nature's Most Powerful Plants

Disclaimer

*The information provided **in The Green Elixir: Unlocking the Health Benefits of Nature's Most Powerful Plants** is intended for educational and informational purposes only. It is not a substitute for **professional medical advice, diagnosis, or treatment**. Always seek the advice of your physician or other qualified healthcare provider with any questions you may have regarding a medical condition **or before incorporating new supplements, plants, or dietary changes** into your routine.*

*While the benefits of the plants discussed in this book are supported by traditional knowledge and emerging scientific studies, individual results may vary. Some **plants may interact with medications or have contraindications** for certain health conditions. Pregnant or nursing women, individuals with allergies, and those managing chronic illnesses should consult a healthcare professional before use.*

*The author and publisher **are not responsible for any adverse effects or consequences** resulting from the use of the information in this book. All readers are encouraged to use their own **discretion and consult with a professional** when applying the knowledge shared herein.*

Contents

Preface

In a world brimming with technological advancements, we often overlook the simple yet profound power of nature. For centuries, indigenous cultures and traditional healers have turned to the plants around them to nurture and heal the body. Plants were, and in many cases still are, the cornerstone of human health and wellness. *The Green Elixir: Unlocking the Health Benefits of Nature's Most Powerful Plants* is my attempt to reconnect with this ancient wisdom and share it with the modern world.

My journey with plant-based healing began with a curiosity about natural remedies, which soon evolved into a passion for discovering how plants can support our physical, mental, and emotional health. Through this book, I hope to inspire you to embrace the plants that have long been valued for their healing properties, and to make them a part of your daily life.

The purpose of this book is simple: to provide you with practical knowledge on how to incorporate nature's most powerful plants into your wellness routine. Whether you're new to plant-based remedies or a seasoned advocate, the information here is designed to be accessible, helpful, and easy to integrate into your lifestyle. From boosting energy to detoxifying the body, supporting immune health, and nourishing the skin, each chapter offers insights into how these plants can transform your health.

This book is not just about facts and figures; it's about inviting nature back into our lives. It's about creating a deeper connection with the earth and unlocking the healing power of plants that have been with us since the dawn of time. I hope this book serves as a guide to living a healthier, more harmonious life by reconnecting with the green elixirs of nature.

Thank you for joining me on this journey. May the plants in these pages offer you the support and healing they have provided to generations before us.

Acknowledgements

Writing this book has been an enriching journey, and I owe a great deal of gratitude to many individuals and communities who have supported and inspired me along the way.

First and foremost, I would like to thank my family and friends for their unwavering support and encouragement throughout this process. Your belief in me, even when self-doubt crept in, has been a constant source of motivation.

A special thank you to the many plant-based health advocates, herbalists, and traditional healers whose wisdom and practices have shaped this book. Although I am not a trained expert in the field, your teachings have inspired me to dive deeper into the world of plants and their profound effects on health.

I would also like to express my appreciation to the researchers and authors whose work on plant medicine laid the foundation for this book. The vast body of knowledge about the benefits of these plants continues to inspire me, and I am grateful for their contributions to the field.

Lastly, I would like to thank you, the reader, for choosing this book. Your interest in exploring the power of nature's plants and integrating them into your life is truly inspiring. I hope you find the knowledge within these pages helpful, and that it empowers you to live a healthier, more connected life.

With sincere gratitude,

Caterinah Muiruri.

Introduction: The Healing Power of Plants

In a world where fast food, artificial supplements, and pharmaceutical solutions often take center stage, it's easy to forget the ancient wisdom that nature has always provided. For centuries, humans have turned to plants for nourishment, healing, and vitality. The healing powers of plants are not new; they've been revered across cultures—from the jungles of Africa to the far reaches of Asia—and their benefits are only now beginning to receive the attention they deserve in modern wellness circles.

In this book, we will explore some of the most powerful plants that nature has given us. These green elixirs—ranging from the mighty moringa tree to the tiny but potent spirulina algae—are packed with essential nutrients, antioxidants, and medicinal properties that support our health in ways we might never have imagined. They offer us an opportunity to reconnect with the natural world and harness the abundance it has to offer.

But why should we care about these plants now, in an age where modern medicine has made incredible advancements? The truth is, while Western medicine has undoubtedly saved countless lives, it's often at the cost of overlooking the simple, yet profound, healing qualities of natural remedies. Our ancestors understood the importance of living in harmony with the earth, and in recent years, many have turned back to these ancient practices as a way to nurture our bodies, minds, and spirits.

This book is not just about providing a list of plants; it's about unlocking their potential in your daily life. Imagine waking up every day with energy that's sustained by the nutrients found in plants like moringa and spirulina. Picture a life where your skin glows, your mind is clear, and your stress levels are at a manageable low—all thanks to the amazing plants we'll explore together.

Each chapter will take you on a journey through one of these remarkable plants, embarking into its nutritional profile, historical significance, and health benefits. You'll learn not only how to incorporate these plants into your diet but also how to appreciate their medicinal properties for holistic wellness. This book is designed to be a guide—one that's easy to follow, practical, and accessible for everyone, whether you're a seasoned herbal enthusiast or someone just starting to explore the world of plant-based health.

By the end of this journey, I hope you'll feel empowered to make these plants an essential part of your life. Whether you're looking to enhance your immune system, detoxify your body, manage stress, or simply feel more vibrant, the green elixirs we'll explore can offer a sustainable and holistic path to wellness. And while modern life may sometimes seem to pull us away from nature, this book will remind you of the quiet power that lies in the earth beneath our feet—waiting for us to discover and embrace it.

 Together, we'll unlock the healing power of nature's most potent plants, and in doing so, we'll bring their wisdom and strength into our daily lives. The journey to better health is simpler than we often realize. All it takes is an open mind, a little curiosity, and the willingness to reconnect with the natural world around us.

Welcome to The Green Elixir. Let's start unlocking the power of plants together.

Chapter 1: The Science of Plant Medicine

Plants have long been used as the cornerstone of medicine in cultures across the globe. From the ancient Egyptians to the Indigenous peoples of North America, plants have been seen not only as food sources but as potent healers, capable of nourishing the body, mind, and spirit. Today, in the face of a rapidly advancing medical system and modern pharmaceuticals, we are rediscovering the profound benefits of nature's pharmacy. But how exactly do plants work their magic?

In this chapter, we'll explore the science behind plant medicine, revealing how plants heal us on a cellular level, why they're so effective, and what makes them a truly sustainable and holistic solution for modern health concerns.

Understanding Phytochemicals: Nature's Secret Ingredients

At the heart of plant medicine lies a diverse group of compounds known as phytochemicals—bioactive substances produced by plants that give them their color, flavor, and resistance to pests. These compounds also offer a multitude of health benefits to humans. There are thousands of different phytochemicals, but the most notable ones that have garnered attention for their medicinal properties include:

Alkaloids: These compounds, which are found in plants like caffeine, tobacco, and morphine, have powerful physiological effects on the human body. In smaller doses, they can act as stimulants, painkillers, or even anti-inflammatory agents.

Flavonoids: Known for their antioxidant and anti-inflammatory properties, flavonoids are found in a variety of fruits, vegetables, and herbs. They play a key role in protecting the body from oxidative stress and chronic disease.

Terpenes: Found in the essential oils of many plants, terpenes are responsible for the aromatic properties of plants like lavender and mint. These compounds also contribute to the anti-inflammatory, antimicrobial, and mood-boosting effects of these plants.

Glycosides: Present in plants like garlic, the glycoside compounds are involved in detoxification processes and support heart health by regulating blood sugar and blood pressure.

Phytochemicals not only help plants survive but also interact with human biology in remarkably beneficial ways. While we have only scratched the surface of their potential, it's these plant compounds that have earned plants their reputation as natural healers.

The Role of Antioxidants and Free Radical Damage

One of the most widely discussed benefits of plants is their high antioxidant content. But what exactly does that mean?

Our cells are constantly exposed to free radicals—unstable molecules that are produced as a byproduct of normal metabolic processes in the body. These free radicals can cause damage to cell membranes, proteins, and even our DNA. This damage, known as oxidative stress, is linked to a range of chronic diseases, including heart disease, diabetes, and cancer.

Plants, however, have developed ways to fight back against oxidative stress, thanks to their high concentrations of antioxidants. Antioxidants are molecules that neutralize free radicals by donating an electron, stabilizing these unstable molecules and preventing further damage. This is one reason why plant-rich diets have been consistently linked to improved overall health.

Take, for example, Moringa, a plant rich in antioxidants like vitamin C and beta-carotene. These antioxidants work together to combat oxidative stress in the body, preventing damage that could lead to chronic illness or even premature aging. In fact, many of the plants featured in this book—spirulina, turmeric, and Matcha—are packed with antioxidants that help reduce oxidative stress and inflammation, protecting your body from the inside out.

Plant Medicine and Our Immune System

Plants don't just help with oxidative stress—they also play a crucial role in supporting our immune system. Many plants contain immune-boosting compounds that enhance the body's natural ability to fight infections, viruses, and bacteria. These compounds often work by stimulating the production of white blood cells, the body's first line of defense against illness.

Take Ashwagandha, for instance. Known for its adaptgenic properties, this plant helps the body respond to stress by regulating the production of cortisol (the stress hormone). But Ashwagandha does more than just reduce stress—it also enhances immune function by increasing the activity of natural killer cells, which are responsible for identifying and destroying pathogens in the body.

Similarly, turmeric contains curcumin, a compound that has been shown to increase the production of white blood cells and activate the immune system's response to infection. The anti-inflammatory properties of curcumin also help reduce the risk of chronic inflammation, which can suppress immune function over time.

Many plants, like neem, possess antiviral and antibacterial properties, offering additional protection against harmful microorganisms. By including these plants in your daily routine, you can help maintain a strong, resilient immune system capable of warding off illnesses.

The Gut-Brain Connection: How Plants Support Mental Health

The relationship between the gut and brain has become an increasingly popular area of research in recent years. Scientists are now discovering just how much our gut health influences our mental health. In fact, around 70% of the body's immune system resides in the gut, which is home to trillions of microorganisms—collectively known as the gut microbiome. These microbes play an essential role in regulating everything from digestion to immune response, and even mood.

Plants are a powerful ally in maintaining a healthy gut microbiome. Many plants, such as baobab and wheatgrass, are rich in prebiotics—non-digestible fibers that feed the beneficial bacteria in your gut. A healthy microbiome supports digestion, enhances nutrient absorption, and even contributes to improved mood and mental clarity.

Moreover, plants like gotu kola have been found to reduce symptoms of anxiety and improve cognitive function. This ancient herb has a long history of use in Ayurvedic medicine for its ability to enhance circulation and promote the growth of new brain cells. The connection between gut health and mental health is one of the most exciting developments in modern wellness, and plants like gotu kola are at the forefront of this research.

Why Plant Medicine is a Sustainable Solution

While pharmaceuticals have their place in modern medicine, they are often associated with side effects, dependency, and environmental costs. The production of synthetic drugs often involves complex chemical processes that can have a negative impact on the environment. Additionally, the overuse of antibiotics and other medications can lead to resistance, creating a need for more powerful drugs.

In contrast, plant-based medicine offers a more sustainable solution. Many plants are renewable, easy to grow, and relatively inexpensive compared to synthetic drugs. The compounds within plants work in harmony with our body's natural systems, offering a gentler, more holistic approach to health. Whether it's using chlorella for detoxification or spirulina for boosting energy, plant medicine is a safe and natural alternative that can support your health without the drawbacks of conventional medicine.

By choosing plant-based solutions, we are not only supporting our bodies but also contributing to the sustainability of the planet. Plants are part of the earth's intricate ecosystem, and by using them responsibly, we can ensure that these natural remedies continue to benefit generations to come.

The Power of Plants in Your Hands

As we move forward into this book, we'll explore some of the most potent plants that you can incorporate into your life. From their nutrient-packed leaves to their powerful medicinal compounds, these plants are more than just food—they are tools for optimal health and wellness. Understanding the science behind plant medicine is the first step in unlocking the incredible benefits these green elixirs have to offer.

In the next chapter, we'll take a closer look at one of the most powerful and versatile plants in the world: moringa. Packed with vitamins, minerals, and antioxidants, this "miracle tree" is just one example of how plants can nourish and heal us. But before we dive into that, take a moment to appreciate the science that makes plant medicine so powerful—and the vast potential that lies in nature's medicine cabinet.

Chapter 2: Moringa – The Miracle Tree

When it comes to plants that pack a punch in terms of nutrition and medicinal properties, moringa stands out as one of the most remarkable. Revered for centuries in traditional medicine, moringa has earned its title as the "Miracle Tree" for its incredible versatility and healing potential. From its nutrient-rich leaves to its potent seeds, moringa has a history of being used to treat everything from malnutrition to inflammation.

In this chapter, we'll explore the science behind Moringa's health benefits, its rich history, and how this humble plant can be incorporated into your daily life to unlock a multitude of wellness benefits.

A Closer Look at Moringa

Moringa oleifera is a fast-growing, drought-resistant tree that's native to the Indian subcontinent. It's a member of the *Moringaceae* family and has been cultivated for over 4,000 years in Africa, Asia, and parts of the Mediterranean. Moringa thrives in dry, arid climates, which makes it a sustainable source of nutrition in regions where food scarcity is a concern. The tree's leaves, pods, flowers, seeds, and roots are all used in various forms of traditional medicine and culinary applications, each offering unique benefits.

Packed with Nutrients

One of the reasons moringa is so highly regarded is its nutritional profile. It is an excellent source of vitamins, minerals, and amino acids, making it a powerful superfood. Here's a breakdown of its nutritional components:

Vitamins: Moringa leaves are a rich source of vitamin A, vitamin C, vitamin E, and several of the B vitamins, including B1 (thiamine), B2 (riboflavin), and B6 (pyridoxine). These vitamins play a crucial role in boosting immunity, protecting the skin, and promoting overall cellular health.

Minerals: Moringa is loaded with essential minerals such as calcium, potassium, magnesium, iron, and zinc. These minerals are critical for bone health, muscle function, hydration, and the proper functioning of enzymes in the body.

Proteins and Amino Acids: Moringa leaves contain all nine essential amino acids, making them a complete protein source. Protein is essential for building and repairing tissues, producing enzymes and hormones, and supporting immune function.

Antioxidants: Moringa is rich in antioxidants like quercetin, chlorogenic acid, and beta-carotene, which help protect the body from oxidative stress and combat free radical damage.

The bioavailability of these nutrients is high, meaning that our body can absorb and utilize them efficiently, making moringa a powerful ally in maintaining good health.

The Medicinal Benefits of Moringa

Moringa's incredible nutritional profile is only the beginning. The plant is also packed with medicinal compounds that have been shown to have a profound effect on various health conditions. Let's explore some of the key benefits:

Anti-Inflammatory Effects: Chronic inflammation is at the root of many common health conditions, including arthritis, heart disease, and diabetes. Moringa contains compounds like flavonoids and polyphenols that act as potent anti-inflammatory agents, helping to reduce swelling and discomfort. Studies have shown that moringa can help alleviate symptoms of inflammatory conditions such as rheumatoid arthritis and inflammatory bowel disease (IBD).

Blood Sugar Regulation: One of the most exciting areas of research on moringa is its potential to help regulate blood sugar levels. Moringa leaves contain compounds that may help lower blood glucose by enhancing insulin sensitivity. This makes moringa a promising natural remedy for individuals dealing with type 2 diabetes or insulin resistance.

Cholesterol Management: Moringa has been found to have a positive impact on cholesterol levels. Its isothiocyanates, a group of sulfur-containing compounds, can help lower both total cholesterol and LDL (bad) cholesterol, reducing the risk of cardiovascular disease. By maintaining a healthy cholesterol profile, moringa can contribute to better heart health.

Detoxification: Moringa has natural detoxifying properties that help rid the body of harmful toxins. The leaves, in particular, are rich in chlorophyll, a compound known for its ability to cleanse the blood and improve liver function. Regular consumption of moringa may support the body's detoxification processes and help purify the blood.

Antimicrobial and Antiviral Properties: Moringa has also been shown to have antibacterial, antifungal, and antiviral properties, making it useful in combating infections. The plant's compounds, including moringin, moringa oil, and benzyl isothiocyanate, help inhibit the growth of harmful bacteria, fungi, and viruses, which can help protect the body from illnesses like colds, flu, and even more serious infections.

Moringa for Mental Clarity and Mood

In addition to its physical health benefits, moringa has also been shown to support mental clarity and mood regulation. The plant contains compounds that have neuroprotective properties, which help improve cognitive function and protect the brain from age-related degeneration.

Moringa's high content of vitamin C and vitamin E also plays a role in protecting the brain from oxidative damage, which can contribute to Alzheimer's disease and other forms of dementia. Moreover, moringa has been found to help reduce symptoms of anxiety and depression, likely due to its ability to balance cortisol levels, the stress hormone, and support the production of serotonin and dopamine, the neurotransmitters responsible for regulating mood.

How to Incorporate Moringa into Your Life

One of the best things about moringa is its versatility. The plant can be consumed in many different forms, each offering unique benefits. Here are some ways to incorporate moringa into your daily routine:

Moringa Powder: The leaves of the moringa tree are often dried and ground into a fine powder. This powder can be added to smoothies, soups, salads, or even sprinkled on top of meals for a nutritional boost. Just one teaspoon of moringa powder can provide a substantial amount of vitamins, minerals, and antioxidants.

Moringa Tea: Moringa tea is a popular way to enjoy the health benefits of this plant. The tea is made by steeping dried moringa leaves in hot water. It's a gentle and soothing way to incorporate moringa into your daily routine, with the added benefit of hydration.

Moringa Capsules: For those who prefer convenience, moringa capsules or tablets are widely available. These capsules offer a concentrated dose of moringa and are easy to incorporate into a busy lifestyle.

Moringa Oil: Moringa oil, extracted from the seeds of the moringa tree, is known for its moisturizing and anti-aging properties. It can be applied topically to the skin to reduce fine lines, nourish the skin, and improve overall skin health. Moringa oil is also a popular ingredient in hair care products due to its ability to promote hair growth and prevent hair loss.

Moringa's Enduring Legacy

Moringa is a true gift from nature, offering a wide array of health benefits backed by centuries of traditional use and modern scientific research. Whether you're seeking to improve your overall health, boost your immune system, manage blood sugar, or support mental clarity, moringa has something to offer. It's more than just a "superfood"—it's a comprehensive solution for better health that can be easily incorporated into your daily life.

In the next chapter, we'll dive into spirulina, another nutrient-dense superfood with its own impressive set of health benefits. But for now, take a moment to appreciate the power of moringa, the Miracle Tree, and all it has to offer for your wellness journey.

Chapter 3: Spirulina – The Blue-Green Powerhouse

When we talk about nutrient-dense superfoods that can truly elevate our health, spirulina stands tall among the best. Known for its vibrant blue-green color, this microscopic alga is packed with an impressive range of nutrients that can boost energy, improve immune function, and support overall wellness. Spirulina is one of the oldest life forms on Earth, dating back over 3.5 billion years, and it has been consumed for centuries for its remarkable health benefits.

In this chapter, we'll dive deep into what makes spirulina so extraordinary, its powerful health benefits, and how you can incorporate this superfood into your daily routine to enhance your vitality and well-being.

What is Spirulina?

Spirulina is a type of cyanobacteria, commonly referred to as blue-green algae, that thrives in both fresh and saltwater environments. This single-celled organism is known for its spiral-shaped structure (hence the name spirulina) and its rich, vibrant color. While spirulina grows naturally in alkaline lakes and ponds, it is also cultivated worldwide for commercial use.

Packed with essential nutrients, spirulina is often considered a "complete food" due to its impressive range of vitamins, minerals, proteins, and antioxidants. In fact, just a small serving of spirulina can provide a significant portion of your daily nutritional needs.

Nutritional Profile of Spirulina

Spirulina is a powerhouse of nutrients, making it an excellent supplement to support health and wellness. Here's a breakdown of some of the key nutrients found in spirulina:

Proteins and Amino Acids: Spirulina is made up of approximately 60-70% protein by weight, which is higher than most plant-based sources. It contains all nine essential amino acids, making it a complete protein source. Amino acids are the building blocks of proteins, which are necessary for building and repairing tissues, enzymes, and hormones in the body.

Vitamins: Spirulina is rich in B vitamins, including B1 (thiamine), B2 (riboflavin), B3 (niacin), and B12 (cobalamin), which play a crucial role in energy production, metabolism, and nervous system health. It's particularly popular among vegans and vegetarians as a non-animal source of B12. Spirulina also contains vitamin A, in the form of beta-carotene, which supports eye health and immune function, as well as vitamin K for healthy blood clotting.

Minerals: Spirulina is an excellent source of iron, which is essential for oxygen transport in the blood, as well as magnesium, which supports muscle function and bone health. Additionally, spirulina provides potassium, calcium, and zinc, which are vital for cardiovascular health, bone strength, and immune function.

Antioxidants: Spirulina is packed with antioxidants, such as phycocyanin, the pigment responsible for its blue-green color. Phycocyanin has powerful anti-inflammatory and antioxidant properties, helping to reduce oxidative stress and prevent cellular damage. Spirulina also contains chlorophyll, which supports detoxification and improves the body's ability to cleanse itself from toxins.

The Health Benefits of Spirulina

Spirulina has gained a reputation as a superfood because of its impressive range of health benefits. Let's explore some of the key ways in which spirulina can improve your well-being:

Boosts Immunity: Spirulina is known to enhance the immune system by stimulating the production of white blood cells and antibodies, which help fight infections. The high levels of vitamin C, beta-carotene, and phycocyanin found in spirulina contribute to its immune-boosting properties, making it a great ally in protecting your body from illnesses.

Increases Energy and Stamina: Due to its high protein content, spirulina can help boost energy levels and increase stamina, making it a great supplement for athletes or those needing an energy pick-me-up. It helps nourish the body's cells with the nutrients they need to function optimally, thus supporting overall vitality.

Supports Detoxification: Spirulina is an excellent detoxifier, primarily due to its rich chlorophyll content. Chlorophyll helps to cleanse the blood, remove toxins, and improve liver function. Spirulina's ability to remove heavy metals and other toxins from the body makes it particularly beneficial for those living in polluted environments or those who have been exposed to toxic substances.

Promotes Healthy Digestion: Spirulina is rich in digestive enzymes and fiber, which can help support gut health. It aids in the breakdown of food and promotes the growth of beneficial gut bacteria, thus improving digestion and nutrient absorption. Spirulina's anti-inflammatory properties may also help soothe the digestive tract and reduce symptoms of conditions like irritable bowel syndrome (IBS).

Helps Control Cholesterol: Studies have shown that spirulina can help lower levels of LDL (bad) cholesterol and triglycerides while increasing HDL (good) cholesterol. This makes spirulina an excellent supplement for supporting heart health and reducing the risk of cardiovascular disease.

Regulates Blood Sugar: Spirulina may help regulate blood sugar levels, which is particularly beneficial for individuals with type 2 diabetes or those at risk of developing the condition. Research has shown that spirulina can reduce blood glucose levels and improve insulin sensitivity, which helps control blood sugar spikes.

Improves Mental Clarity and Mood: Spirulina's rich content of B vitamins and antioxidants can help boost brain function and improve mental clarity. The algae have been shown to reduce symptoms of depression, anxiety, and stress, thanks to its ability to regulate cortisol levels and support neurotransmitter function. Additionally, spirulina's rich magnesium content helps promote relaxation and reduce nervous tension.

Incorporating Spirulina into Your Diet

Spirulina is available in a variety of forms, including powder, tablets, and capsules. Here are some simple ways to add this blue-green powerhouse to your daily routine:

Spirulina Powder: The most versatile form of spirulina, spirulina powder can be added to smoothies, juices, soups, or even sprinkled over salads. Start with a small dose (about 1 teaspoon) and gradually increase the amount as your body gets used to it. The powder has a strong, earthy flavor, which may take some getting used to, but it's an easy way to enjoy all the benefits of spirulina.

Spirulina Tablets or Capsules: If you prefer convenience, spirulina is widely available in tablet or capsule form. This allows for an easy, on-the-go supplement that requires no preparation. You can take it as a daily supplement with water or mix it into a smoothie.

Spirulina in Energy Bars: Many health food brands now offer energy bars or snacks that include spirulina as one of the main ingredients. These are a great way to add spirulina to your diet while satisfying your hunger.

Spirulina Smoothies: Add a teaspoon or two of spirulina powder to your favorite smoothie. It blends well with fruits like bananas, berries, or pineapples and can be easily masked by the natural sweetness of the fruit. You can also add other superfoods like moringa or chia seeds for an added nutritional boost.

Precautions and Considerations

While spirulina is generally considered safe for most people, it's important to keep a few things in mind:

Quality: Since spirulina is grown in water, it's important to source it from reputable suppliers to ensure it's free from contaminants, such as heavy metals or toxins. Always choose spirulina that is certified organic and has been tested for purity.

Pregnancy and Breastfeeding: Pregnant or breastfeeding women should consult with their healthcare provider before using spirulina, just to be safe.

Allergic Reactions: Some individuals may experience allergic reactions to spirulina, including skin rashes or digestive discomfort. Start with a small amount to see how your body reacts.

Spirulina's Lasting Impact on Health

Spirulina is truly a gift from the ocean, offering a wide range of health benefits that can support every aspect of your well-being. From boosting energy and immunity to improving digestion and heart health, spirulina is a versatile superfood that deserves a place in your diet. Whether you're an athlete, a busy professional, or someone looking to improve your overall health, spirulina is a powerhouse supplement that can help you achieve your wellness goals.

In the next chapter, we'll explore another nutrient-dense superfood—chlorella—and how it can further support your health. But for now, take a moment to appreciate the vitality and wellness that spirulina brings to your life.

Chapter 4: Chlorella – The Green Powerhouse of Detoxification

In the world of superfoods, few are as revered for their detoxifying properties as chlorella. These tiny green algae have a remarkable ability to cleanse the body, detoxify heavy metals, and improve immune function. A powerhouse of essential nutrients, chlorella is quickly gaining attention for its ability to support overall health, vitality, and well-being.

In this chapter, we'll explore the incredible health benefits of chlorella, its nutritional profile, and how to incorporate this green gem into your diet for maximum effect. Whether you're seeking to detoxify, boost your energy, or enhance your immune system, chlorella might just be the secret weapon you need.

What is Chlorella?

Chlorella is a single-celled green algae that grows in freshwater environments. It is rich in chlorophyll, the pigment responsible for its deep green color, and is known for its remarkable ability to promote detoxification and support the body's natural healing processes. Chlorella has been consumed for thousands of years, particularly in Japan and other parts of Asia, where it has been used for its medicinal and health benefits.

What makes chlorella truly unique is its cell wall. Unlike most other algae, chlorella has a tough, indigestible cell wall that, once broken down, releases its full nutritional potential. This cell wall is often processed before consumption to ensure that the body can fully absorb its nutrients, which is why chlorella supplements are often sold in powder or tablet form.

Nutritional Profile of Chlorella

Chlorella is one of the most nutrient-dense foods on the planet, offering an impressive array of vitamins, minerals, and other bioactive compounds that support overall health. Here's a breakdown of some of the most important nutrients found in chlorella:

Proteins and Amino Acids: Chlorella contains about 50-60% protein by weight, making it an excellent plant-based source of protein. The protein found in chlorella is of high quality, containing all nine essential amino acids. This makes chlorella an excellent choice for vegetarians, vegans, or anyone looking to increase their protein intake without consuming animal products.

Vitamins: Chlorella is an excellent source of B vitamins, including B1 (thiamine), B2 (riboflavin), B3 (niacin), B6 (pyridoxine), and B12 (cobalamin). These vitamins play a crucial role in energy production, metabolism, and overall cell function. Chlorella is particularly valued as a natural source of vitamin B12, which is important for vegans who may struggle to get enough B12 from plant-based sources. Additionally, chlorella contains vitamin A, which supports immune health and vision, and vitamin C, which aids in collagen production and protects the body from oxidative stress.

Minerals: Chlorella is rich in essential minerals, including iron, which is important for oxygen transport in the blood, magnesium, which supports muscle function and nerve health, and calcium, which is essential for bone health. It also contains zinc, which plays a key role in immune function and cell growth.

Chlorophyll: One of chlorella's most notable features is its high chlorophyll content. Chlorophyll is a powerful antioxidant and has detoxifying properties, helping to cleanse the blood and remove toxins from the body. It also supports liver health, which plays a crucial role in detoxification.

Omega-3 Fatty Acids: Chlorella contains omega-3 fatty acids, which are essential fats that support brain function, reduce inflammation, and promote heart health. While chlorella is not as high in omega-3s as fatty fish or certain seeds, it can still provide a beneficial dose of these important fats.

Carotenoids: Chlorella contains several carotenoids, including lutein and zeaxanthin, which are known to support eye health and protect against age-related macular degeneration.

The Health Benefits of Chlorella

Chlorella is a truly remarkable superfood, offering an array of health benefits that extend far beyond basic nutrition. Here are some of the most notable ways chlorella can support your health and well-being:

Detoxification: Chlorella is perhaps best known for its powerful detoxifying properties. It has the ability to bind to heavy metals, such as mercury, lead, and cadmium, and help remove them from the body. This makes chlorella an excellent supplement for individuals who have been exposed to environmental toxins or those seeking to support their body's natural detoxification processes. The high chlorophyll content in chlorella also helps to cleanse the liver, which is the body's primary detox organ.

Boosts Immune Function: Chlorella has been shown to enhance immune function by stimulating the production of white blood cells, which are responsible for fighting infections. The vitamins, minerals, and antioxidants found in chlorella help to strengthen the immune system, making it easier for the body to defend against illness and disease.

Improves Digestion and Gut Health: Chlorella is a natural source of fiber and enzymes that support digestive health. The fiber in chlorella helps to promote regular bowel movements, reduce constipation, and support healthy gut bacteria. Chlorella's anti-inflammatory properties also help to soothe the digestive tract and reduce symptoms of irritable bowel syndrome (IBS), bloating, and gas.

Supports Heart Health: Chlorella has been shown to help lower blood pressure and reduce cholesterol levels, which can help protect against cardiovascular disease. Its rich content of omega-3 fatty acids and chlorophyll work together to support healthy circulation, reduce inflammation, and maintain healthy blood vessels.

Enhances Skin Health: The antioxidants found in chlorella, particularly vitamin C, beta-carotene, and chlorophyll, help protect the skin from oxidative stress and premature aging. Chlorella also supports collagen production, which is essential for maintaining skin elasticity and reducing the appearance of wrinkles. Its anti-inflammatory properties can also help reduce acne and other skin irritations.

Promotes Healthy Blood Sugar Levels: Some studies have shown that chlorella can help regulate blood sugar levels, making it beneficial for individuals with type 2 diabetes or those at risk of developing the condition. Chlorella helps improve insulin sensitivity, which aids in better blood sugar control.

Enhances Energy and Vitality: Chlorella's high nutrient content helps nourish the body and boost energy levels. The B vitamins in chlorella are particularly beneficial for converting food into energy, while its rich protein and amino acid content support muscle recovery and stamina. Regular consumption of chlorella may result in increased vitality and an improved sense of overall well-being.

Incorporating Chlorella into Your Diet

Like spirulina, chlorella is available in various forms, including powder, tablets, and capsules. Here are some of the easiest ways to include chlorella in your daily routine:

Chlorella Powder: Chlorella powder is incredibly versatile and can be added to smoothies, juices, or even soups. Start with a small dose (about 1 teaspoon) and gradually increase the amount as your body adjusts. The powder has a strong, earthy flavor, so it pairs well with other greens, fruits, and citrus to mask the taste.

Chlorella Tablets or Capsules: If you prefer convenience, chlorella tablets or capsules are an easy way to get your daily dose of this green superfood. These are available in a variety of dosages, and you can take them with water or combine them with a smoothie or meal.

Chlorella in Energy Bars: Many health food brands offer energy bars and snacks that incorporate chlorella. These are perfect for an on-the-go detox or as a midday energy boost.

Chlorella Smoothies: Adding chlorella powder to your smoothie is an easy and delicious way to get your greens. Combine it with fruits like bananas, berries, and citrus for a nutrient-packed, detoxifying drink.

Precautions and Considerations

While chlorella is generally safe for most people, it's important to keep a few things in mind:

Quality: As with spirulina, ensure that you choose chlorella from a reputable source. The cell walls of chlorella must be properly broken down to make the nutrients bioavailable, so look for high-quality, broken-cell-wall chlorella.

Pregnancy and Breastfeeding: Consult with your healthcare provider before taking chlorella if you are pregnant or breastfeeding, as its detoxifying effects may be too intense during these stages.

Allergic Reactions: Some individuals may experience allergic reactions to chlorella, including digestive discomfort or skin rashes. Start with a small amount and monitor your body's response.

Embrace the Green Detox Power

Chlorella is a powerful superfood that supports detoxification, boosts immune function, enhances digestion, and promotes overall health. Whether you're looking to cleanse your body from toxins, improve skin health, or enhance your energy levels, chlorella offers a multitude of benefits to help you achieve your wellness goals.

Chapter 8: Ginkgo Biloba - Unlocking Mental Clarity and Cognitive Health

What is Ginkgo Biloba?

Ginkgo Biloba, often referred to simply as ginkgo, is one of the oldest living tree species, with a history spanning over 200 million years. Known for its distinctive fan-shaped leaves, this tree has been a symbol of resilience and longevity in traditional medicine. Ginkgo Biloba is celebrated primarily for its remarkable effects on brain function, earning its place as a popular supplement for enhancing cognitive health.

The medicinal use of ginkgo dates back thousands of years in Traditional Chinese Medicine (TCM), where it was revered for its ability to improve circulation, support brain health, and treat a variety of ailments. Today, ginkgo biloba is widely used as a supplement, often found in capsules, extracts, or teas. Its cognitive benefits are particularly sought after in today's fast-paced world, where mental clarity, memory, and focus are in high demand.

Health Benefits of Ginkgo Biloba

1. Improved Memory and Cognitive Function

Ginkgo biloba is most widely known for its ability to enhance memory, focus, and overall cognitive performance. The active compounds in ginkgo, particularly flavonoids and terpenoids, have been shown to improve blood flow to the brain, which may help boost memory and cognitive function, particularly in older adults. Research suggests that ginkgo can be beneficial for those suffering from age-related cognitive decline, including conditions like Alzheimer's disease and dementia.

Studies have indicated that ginkgo biloba can increase the uptake of glucose and oxygen in brain cells, essential for their energy needs and function. As a result, individuals who take ginkgo report improvements in their ability to concentrate, think more clearly, and remember important details.

2. Enhanced Mental Clarity and Focus

Whether you're studying, working on a complex project, or simply need to stay sharp throughout the day, ginkgo may be a helpful ally. The improved blood circulation it promotes ensures that your brain receives the nutrients it needs to function optimally, thus enhancing mental clarity. Many people report feeling more alert, focused, and clear-headed after incorporating ginkgo into their routine, making it a popular supplement for students and professionals alike.

3. Boosting Circulation and Heart Health

Ginkgo biloba plays an important role in promoting healthy circulation throughout the body. By improving blood flow, especially to the extremities, ginkgo can help alleviate symptoms of poor circulation, such as cold hands and feet. It has also been linked to a reduction in high blood pressure, which is a major risk factor for heart disease.

The antioxidants in ginkgo, including flavonoids and terpenoids, also protect blood vessels from oxidative damage, contributing to arterial health and reducing the risk of cardiovascular diseases like stroke and heart attack. This makes ginkgo biloba a powerful herb for maintaining overall heart health.

4. Relieving Anxiety and Stress

In addition to supporting brain health, ginkgo has been found to have potential anxiolytic (anxiety-reducing) effects. Research shows that ginkgo can help reduce symptoms of anxiety by modulating certain brain chemicals, such as serotonin and dopamine, which play crucial roles in regulating mood and stress levels.

For those struggling with stress and anxiety, incorporating ginkgo biloba into their wellness regimen may help foster a sense of calm and reduce the emotional burden of daily challenges.

5. Protecting Eye Health

Ginkgo biloba may also have a positive effect on eye health, particularly in individuals with age-related macular degeneration and glaucoma. The improved blood circulation that ginkgo promotes can help ensure the eyes receive adequate oxygen and nutrients, supporting healthy vision and possibly preventing further degeneration.

Some studies have also shown that ginkgo can protect against oxidative damage in the eyes, which is a key factor in the development of cataracts and other age-related eye conditions.

6. Improved Mood and Mental Well-being

Along with its ability to reduce anxiety, ginkgo biloba has been linked to improvements in mood. By enhancing circulation and supporting overall brain function, ginkgo may contribute to a more positive outlook and a greater sense of well-being. This makes it particularly helpful for individuals who may be dealing with seasonal affective disorder (SAD) or other mood-related conditions.

How to Incorporate Ginkgo Biloba into Your Routine?

Ginkgo biloba is available in a variety of forms, including capsules, tablets, liquid extracts, and teas. The most common method of consumption is through standardized capsules or tablets, which ensure that you are getting a consistent and effective dose. The typical dosage ranges from 120 to 240 milligrams per day, divided into two or three doses.

Tea: If you prefer a more natural approach, ginkgo biloba tea is a great option. Simply steep a ginkgo biloba leaf in hot water for several minutes. While it may not be as concentrated as capsules or extracts, it can still offer some benefits to help improve circulation and mental clarity.

Extracts and Tinctures: For those looking for a more potent dose, ginkgo biloba extracts and tinctures are an effective way to get the full benefits. These concentrated forms of ginkgo can be added to water or juice for easy consumption.

When incorporating ginkgo into your daily routine, it's important to choose high-quality supplements from reputable brands that ensure their products are free from contaminants. Be sure to start with a lower dose to assess your body's response, and gradually increase it if necessary.

Precautions and Side Effects

While ginkgo biloba is generally considered safe for most people, there are some precautions and side effects to keep in mind:

1. Blood Thinning: Ginkgo has natural blood-thinning properties, which can be beneficial for improving circulation but may pose risks for individuals taking blood thinners (such as warfarin or aspirin). If you are on any medication to manage blood clotting, consult with your healthcare provider before using ginkgo biloba.

2. Potential for Allergic Reactions: Though rare, some individuals may experience an allergic reaction to ginkgo biloba. Symptoms can include rash, itching, or swelling. If you experience any of these symptoms, discontinue use immediately and seek medical advice.

3. Gastrointestinal Discomfort: In some cases, ginkgo can cause mild gastrointestinal discomfort, including nausea, stomach cramps, or diarrhea. If you experience these side effects, consider reducing your dosage or switching to a different form of ginkgo (e.g., from capsule to tea).

4. Pregnancy and Breastfeeding: As with many herbs, ginkgo biloba is not recommended during pregnancy or breastfeeding unless specifically advised by your healthcare provider. The effects of ginkgo on fetal development and breastfeeding are not well-established.

5. Interactions with Medications: Ginkgo biloba can interact with various medications, particularly those for diabetes, high blood pressure, and antidepressants. Always consult your doctor before introducing ginkgo to your regimen, especially if you are taking any prescription medications.

Conclusion

Ginkgo biloba is a time-tested natural remedy that can help improve mental clarity, boost cognitive function, and promote overall brain health. Whether you're looking to sharpen your focus, reduce anxiety, or protect your eyes and heart, ginkgo offers a powerful solution. By enhancing circulation, improving nutrient delivery to the brain, and offering potent antioxidant protection, ginkgo biloba remains a valuable tool in maintaining optimal cognitive function and mental well-being as you age.

Stay tuned for the next chapter, where we will explore Turmeric and its anti-inflammatory and healing benefits. Ginkgo is just one part of the puzzle when it comes to natural health, and there are many more powerful herbs and superfoods to explore on your wellness journey.

Chapter 9: Turmeric - The Golden Spice for Healing and Inflammation

What is Turmeric?

Turmeric, often called the "golden spice," is a vibrant yellow-orange root that comes from the Curcuma longa plant. It has been used for thousands of years in Traditional Indian Medicine (Ayurveda) and Traditional Chinese Medicine (TCM) as a powerful healing herb due to its rich anti-inflammatory, antioxidant, and antimicrobial properties. The active compound responsible for much of its healing power is curcumin, a bright yellow pigment that gives turmeric its distinctive color.

Turmeric is not only a staple in culinary dishes, especially in Indian cuisine, but it has also become increasingly popular in the wellness world for its impressive health benefits. From promoting joint health to supporting brain function, turmeric's versatility makes it one of the most sought-after superfoods globally.

Health Benefits of Turmeric

1. Anti-Inflammatory Power

Chronic inflammation is linked to numerous health issues, including heart disease, arthritis, diabetes, and even cancer. Turmeric's primary active ingredient, curcumin, is known for its potent anti-inflammatory properties. It works by blocking certain enzymes and proteins that contribute to the inflammatory process. By reducing inflammation in the body, turmeric can help prevent or manage conditions related to chronic inflammation, such as osteoarthritis and rheumatoid arthritis.

Studies have shown that curcumin is as effective as some anti-inflammatory drugs, but with fewer side effects, making it a safer option for long-term use.

2. Pain Relief and Joint Health

Turmeric is particularly effective for individuals dealing with joint pain, stiffness, and arthritis. Its anti-inflammatory properties can reduce swelling, relieve pain, and improve mobility. For those with conditions like osteoarthritis, taking turmeric supplements or consuming turmeric regularly can help decrease pain and enhance flexibility. Many people turn to turmeric as a natural alternative to NSAIDs (nonsteroidal anti-inflammatory drugs), which can have side effects such as stomach irritation and kidney damage with prolonged use.

Studies suggest that turmeric can significantly improve joint function and reduce the symptoms of chronic pain associated with conditions like rheumatoid arthritis and fibromyalgia.

3. Supports Brain Function

Curcumin has been shown to cross the blood-brain barrier, a protective mechanism that shields the brain from harmful substances. Once inside, it helps increase levels of a crucial brain hormone called brain-derived neurotrophic factor (BDNF). BDNF plays a key role in brain function, particularly in terms of memory, learning, and cognitive performance. Low levels of BDNF have been associated with depression, Alzheimer's disease, and other neurodegenerative conditions.

By boosting BDNF levels, turmeric may help enhance brain function and even reduce the risk of brain diseases. Studies have found that people who regularly consume turmeric have better memory and cognitive function, especially as they age.

4. Antioxidant Properties and Cancer Prevention

Turmeric is a powerhouse of antioxidants, which help neutralize free radicals in the body—unstable molecules that can damage cells and lead to chronic diseases and aging. Curcumin is one of the most powerful antioxidants in nature, and it not only fights oxidative stress but also enhances the body's own antioxidant defense systems.

Numerous studies have suggested that turmeric may play a role in cancer prevention. Curcumin has been shown to inhibit the growth of cancer cells, slow the spread of tumors, and even promote the death of cancer cells. While turmeric is not a cure for cancer, its ability to reduce inflammation and oxidative stress can certainly lower the risk of developing certain types of cancer, particularly in the colon, breast, and prostate.

5. Digestive Health

Turmeric has been used for centuries as a digestive aid in various traditional medicine systems. It can help stimulate the production of bile, which aids in digestion and the breakdown of fats. This makes it an excellent choice for individuals dealing with bloating, indigestion, or irritable bowel syndrome (IBS). Turmeric is also known to have antimicrobial properties, which can help combat gut infections and improve overall gut health.

For those struggling with digestive issues or discomfort after meals, adding turmeric to their diet can significantly improve gut health, promote smoother digestion, and reduce symptoms of acid reflux.

6. Heart Health and Cholesterol Control

The anti-inflammatory and antioxidant properties of turmeric also play a significant role in promoting heart health. Chronic inflammation is a key contributor to atherosclerosis (hardening of the arteries), a condition that can lead to heart attacks or strokes. By reducing inflammation and oxidative stress, turmeric can help keep your arteries flexible and free from plaque buildup.

In addition, turmeric can help regulate cholesterol levels by increasing the production of HDL (good cholesterol) while reducing LDL (bad cholesterol). This can improve overall cardiovascular health and reduce the risk of developing heart disease.

7. Skin Health and Healing

Turmeric has been used for centuries as a skin treatment for its ability to promote healing and treat various skin conditions. Its anti-inflammatory and antimicrobial properties help reduce redness, swelling, and irritation caused by conditions such as eczema, psoriasis, and acne.

When applied topically or consumed internally, turmeric can also promote the healing of wounds and reduce the appearance of scars. The anti-inflammatory effects can also reduce the appearance of dark spots and improve the overall texture of the skin.

8. Mood and Mental Health

Turmeric may offer significant benefits for individuals struggling with mood disorders such as depression. Curcumin has been shown to increase the levels of serotonin and dopamine—two neurotransmitters that play crucial roles in regulating mood and mental well-being. In some studies, curcumin supplementation has been shown to improve symptoms of depression, with results comparable to conventional antidepressants.

Regular consumption of turmeric can support better mood regulation, reduce feelings of anxiety, and promote a sense of overall well-being.

How to Incorporate Turmeric into Your Routine

Turmeric is incredibly versatile and can be used in various forms to enjoy its health benefits. Here are some common ways to incorporate it into your daily routine:

1. Golden Milk (Turmeric Latte): A popular way to enjoy turmeric is by making golden milk, which is a warm drink made with turmeric, milk (or plant-based milk), honey, and black pepper. The addition of black pepper is crucial, as it enhances the absorption of curcumin in the body by up to 2,000%.

2. Turmeric Supplements: If you're looking for a more concentrated dose of turmeric, you can take turmeric supplements in the form of capsules or tablets. Be sure to choose a supplement that contains bioavailable curcumin and is standardized for optimal potency.

3. Smoothies: Add turmeric powder to your morning smoothie for a flavorful, health-boosting addition. Pair

it with fruits, vegetables, and healthy fats to enhance absorption.

4. Curry Dishes: Turmeric is a key ingredient in many curry recipes, which is why it's so prevalent in Indian cuisine. You can add it to stews, soups, rice dishes, and even roasted vegetables for a flavorful twist.

5. Turmeric Tea: Steep fresh turmeric root in hot water to make a soothing turmeric tea. You can also add ginger and honey to enhance its anti-inflammatory and antioxidant effects.

Precautions and Side Effects

While turmeric is generally safe for most people when consumed in moderate amounts, there are some precautions to consider:

1. Stomach Upset: High doses of turmeric or curcumin supplements can cause digestive upset, including nausea, stomach cramps, or diarrhea. It's best to start with a small dose and gradually increase it.

2. Blood Thinning: Turmeric has natural blood-thinning properties, which can interfere with blood-thinning medications like warfarin. If you are on such medications, consult with your doctor before using turmeric regularly.

3. Pregnancy and Breastfeeding: Turmeric is considered safe in food amounts during pregnancy, but

high doses or concentrated forms, such as supplements, should be avoided unless advised by your healthcare provider.

4. Gallbladder Issues: People with gallstones or other gallbladder conditions should avoid high doses of turmeric, as it may stimulate the gallbladder and cause discomfort.

Turmeric is a potent, natural remedy that can benefit nearly every aspect of your health. From its powerful anti-inflammatory effects to its ability to support brain function, improve heart health, and enhance mood, turmeric truly deserves its title as a superfood. With its versatility in the kitchen and as a supplement, it's easy to incorporate this golden spice into your daily routine.

In the next chapter, we'll explore Ashwagandha, a powerful adaptogen known for its stress-reducing properties and ability to improve overall vitality. Stay tuned as we continue our journey into the world of healing herbs and superfoods!

Chapter 10: Ashwagandha - The Adaptogen for Stress and Vitality

What is Ashwagandha?

Ashwagandha, scientifically known as *Withania somnifera,* is a medicinal herb that has been used for over 3,000 years in Ayurvedic medicine to promote longevity, reduce stress, and increase overall vitality. Known as an adaptogen, ashwagandha helps the body adapt to physical and emotional stress, making it a powerful ally for those struggling with anxiety, fatigue, and mental burnout.

The name "ashwagandha" comes from the Sanskrit word "ashwa", meaning horse, and "gandha", meaning smell, referring to the strong scent of the root. Traditionally, ashwagandha is revered for its ability to rejuvenate the body and restore energy, making it an essential part of herbal medicine across various cultures, particularly in India and other parts of Southeast Asia.

Health Benefits of Ashwagandha

1. Stress Reduction and Adaptogenic Effects

One of ashwagandha's most well-known benefits is its ability to act as an adaptogen. Adaptogens are natural substances that help the body respond to stress by regulating the HPA (hypothalamic-pituitary-adrenal) axis and balancing the release of cortisol, the body's primary stress hormone. Chronic stress leads to elevated cortisol levels, which can result in symptoms like anxiety, fatigue, and irritability. By normalizing cortisol levels, ashwagandha helps mitigate these effects, promoting a calmer, more relaxed state.

Several clinical studies have shown that ashwagandha significantly reduces cortisol levels, which, in turn, helps improve stress resilience. People who experience high levels of stress in their daily lives, such as those with demanding jobs or personal challenges, can benefit from incorporating ashwagandha into their wellness routine to manage stress more effectively.

2. Anxiety and Depression Relief

Ashwagandha has long been used in Ayurvedic medicine to help calm the nervous system and alleviate symptoms of anxiety and depression. Studies show that ashwagandha's ability to reduce cortisol not only calms stress but also helps improve mood and reduce feelings of anxiety. Additionally, the herb has antidepressant-like effects, as it supports the production of serotonin and dopamine, neurotransmitters responsible for mood regulation.

Research has demonstrated that individuals with chronic anxiety who supplement with ashwagandha experience a significant reduction in symptoms, sometimes comparable to traditional anti-anxiety medications. Ashwagandha's calming effects make it a wonderful alternative for those looking for natural solutions to anxiety without the side effects of pharmaceuticals.

3. Boosting Energy and Reducing Fatigue

Ashwagandha is also known for its ability to combat fatigue and improve overall energy levels. Its rejuvenating effects on the body help restore vitality, particularly in individuals who feel physically or mentally drained from stress or overwork. Unlike stimulants like caffeine, ashwagandha works by restoring balance within the body's systems, ensuring sustained energy without the jitters or crashes.

It also supports the adrenal glands, which are responsible for managing the body's response to stress. By ensuring that the adrenal glands function optimally, ashwagandha helps reduce fatigue and enhances overall physical performance. This makes it a great choice for people dealing with chronic fatigue syndrome or those simply looking to improve their energy levels.

4. Improved Sleep Quality

Sleep disturbances, such as insomnia or restlessness, are common in individuals dealing with chronic stress, anxiety, or depression. Ashwagandha helps promote more restful, deeper sleep by reducing anxiety and balancing cortisol levels, both of which are major contributors to poor sleep quality. In clinical studies, participants who took ashwagandha before bed reported improved sleep quality and an increased sense of refreshment upon waking.

In addition to supporting better sleep, ashwagandha has been shown to reduce the time it takes to fall asleep and increase overall sleep duration. For those who struggle with insomnia or disrupted sleep patterns, ashwagandha can be a natural and effective solution.

5. Enhancing Cognitive Function and Brain Health

Ashwagandha has been shown to have neuroprotective effects, which help support brain function, memory, and cognition. The herb enhances the production of acetylcholine, a neurotransmitter involved in learning and memory processes, thereby improving cognitive performance.

It also helps reduce oxidative stress and inflammation in the brain, which are believed to contribute to neurodegenerative diseases such as Alzheimer's and Parkinson's. By reducing the damage to brain cells, ashwagandha plays a protective role in preserving cognitive function over time.

For individuals who experience mental fatigue or cognitive decline, ashwagandha can help sharpen memory and enhance concentration, making it an excellent herb for boosting overall mental clarity.

6. Boosting Immune Function

Ashwagandha is known for its immunomodulatory effects, meaning it helps regulate and strengthen the immune system. It has been shown to enhance the activity of white blood cells, which are essential for fighting off infections. Regular use of ashwagandha can help improve the body's ability to ward off common colds, flu, and other infections.

The herb also promotes the production of interferon, a protein that plays a crucial role in protecting cells from viral infections. Ashwagandha's ability to boost immunity makes it an excellent addition to any wellness routine, especially during flu season or periods of stress, when immune function can be compromised.

7. Supporting Hormonal Balance and Fertility

Ashwagandha is often used to support hormonal balance, particularly for individuals dealing with thyroid issues or adrenal dysfunction. It has been shown to support thyroid hormone production, which is critical for metabolism, energy production, and overall health. People with hypothyroidism (an underactive thyroid) may benefit from ashwagandha's ability to stimulate the production of thyroid hormones.

In addition, ashwagandha is beneficial for improving fertility. Studies suggest that ashwagandha can increase sperm count and motility in men, making it a natural option for couples struggling with infertility. For women, ashwagandha can help regulate the menstrual cycle, improve ovulation, and support overall reproductive health.

8. Supporting Heart Health

Ashwagandha is believed to have a positive effect on heart health by reducing cholesterol and improving blood circulation. It helps reduce the levels of LDL (bad cholesterol) while increasing the production of HDL (good cholesterol), leading to a healthier lipid profile.

Additionally, ashwagandha's anti-inflammatory properties help reduce the risk of atherosclerosis (hardening of the arteries), a condition that can lead to heart attacks or strokes. Regular consumption of ashwagandha may therefore help reduce overall cardiovascular risk.

How to Incorporate Ashwagandha into Your Routine

Ashwagandha can be consumed in several forms to suit your lifestyle:

1. Ashwagandha Powder: You can add ashwagandha powder to smoothies, tea, or warm milk (also known as golden milk). It's a versatile way to consume the herb daily.

2. Ashwagandha Capsules or Tablets: For those who prefer a more concentrated form of the herb, ashwagandha supplements in capsule or tablet form are widely available. Be sure to choose a high-quality supplement that provides the correct dosage.

3. Ashwagandha Tea: Ashwagandha can also be brewed into a tea. Many herbal tea blends contain ashwagandha, and you can combine it with other relaxing herbs such as chamomile or lemon balm for a soothing bedtime ritual.

4. Ashwagandha Tinctures or Extracts: For those looking for a fast-acting solution, ashwagandha tinctures or liquid extracts are an excellent option. These provide a concentrated dose and are absorbed more quickly than powders or capsules.

5. Ashwagandha in Cooking: Ashwagandha can also be added to soups, stews, and curries, especially in traditional Ayurvedic recipes. Its earthy taste blends well with both sweet and savory dishes.

Precautions and Side Effects

While ashwagandha is generally considered safe for most people, there are a few considerations to keep in mind:

1. Pregnancy and Breastfeeding: Pregnant women should avoid using ashwagandha, as it may cause uterine contractions. It is also recommended to consult a healthcare provider before using ashwagandha while breastfeeding.

2. Thyroid Conditions: Individuals with hyperthyroidism (an overactive thyroid) should consult a healthcare provider before using ashwagandha, as it can stimulate thyroid hormone production.

3. Blood Pressure and Blood Sugar: Ashwagandha may have a mild effect on blood pressure and blood sugar levels. People on medication for these conditions should consult their doctor before adding ashwagandha to their routine.

4. Side Effects: Some people may experience mild side effects such as digestive upset, headache, or drowsiness, especially when taking large doses. Starting with a smaller dose and gradually increasing it can help minimize these effects. If you experience any severe side effects such as dizziness, nausea, or allergic reactions, discontinue use and consult a healthcare provider.

Recommended Dosage

The appropriate dosage of ashwagandha can vary based on individual health needs and the form in which it is consumed. However, here are some general guidelines:

Ashwagandha Powder: Typically, 1-2 teaspoons (approximately 3-6 grams) of ashwagandha powder can be taken daily. It can be mixed into a smoothie, tea, or warm milk.

Ashwagandha Capsules/Tablets: Standard dosages for ashwagandha supplements range from 300 mg to 500 mg taken once or twice daily, though higher doses may be used under medical supervision.

Ashwagandha Tinctures: A typical dose for tinctures ranges from 1 to 2 teaspoons (5-10 mL) per day.

It's always best to start with the lowest recommended dosage and increase gradually, depending on how your body responds.

Conclusion

Ashwagandha is a powerful herb with a long history of use in traditional medicine. Its wide range of benefits—from reducing stress and anxiety to boosting energy, supporting immune function, and enhancing cognitive performance—makes it a valuable addition to anyone's wellness routine. Whether you're looking to enhance your resilience to stress, improve your sleep, or boost your overall vitality, ashwagandha can be an effective, natural solution.

As with any supplement or herbal remedy, it's essential to use ashwagandha responsibly, consult with a healthcare provider if you have existing health conditions, and ensure that you're purchasing high-quality products. By incorporating ashwagandha into your daily life, you're supporting your body's ability to adapt to stress, maintain balance, and thrive.

Chapter 12: Ginger - The Root of Vitality and Wellness

What is Ginger?

Ginger, scientifically known as *Zingiber officinale,* is a flowering plant native to Southeast Asia, with its roots (or rhizomes) being the most commonly used part for both culinary and medicinal purposes. Known for its distinctive spicy flavor, ginger has been utilized for thousands of years in traditional medicine, particularly in Chinese and Ayurvedic practices. It has gained worldwide popularity as a key ingredient in cooking and as a supplement for its numerous health benefits.

Ginger contains a variety of bioactive compounds, such as gingerol, shogaol, and zingiberene, which are responsible for its medicinal properties. These compounds give ginger its distinctive taste and contribute to its healing capabilities. Whether fresh, dried, or powdered, ginger has a long history of supporting the body in numerous ways—from aiding digestion to alleviating nausea and inflammation.

Health Benefits of Ginger

1. Supports Digestive Health

Ginger has long been used as a remedy for digestive issues such as indigestion, nausea, and bloating. One of ginger's most significant benefits is its ability to aid in the digestive process. It enhances the production of gastric juices, which helps with the breakdown and absorption of nutrients from food.

Ginger has also been shown to stimulate peristalsis, the movement of food and waste through the intestines, helping prevent constipation and promoting regular bowel movements. Additionally, it can ease discomfort from indigestion by relaxing the muscles in the gastrointestinal tract, allowing food to pass more easily.

For individuals experiencing nausea—whether due to motion sickness, morning sickness during pregnancy, or chemotherapy—ginger has been shown to significantly reduce symptoms. It works by enhancing the movement of food and fluids in the stomach, preventing them from stagnating and causing nausea.

2. Anti-Inflammatory and Pain Relief

Ginger is an excellent natural remedy for those suffering from inflammatory conditions such as arthritis, rheumatoid arthritis, and osteoarthritis. It has potent anti-inflammatory properties that work by inhibiting pro-inflammatory molecules and enzymes, reducing joint pain, swelling, and stiffness. Ginger can be particularly effective when taken regularly as part of an overall treatment plan for managing chronic inflammation.

Studies have shown that ginger can reduce the pain and discomfort associated with muscle soreness and joint pain by blocking the production of inflammatory compounds in the body. It is often used by athletes to relieve post-workout muscle stiffness or anyone suffering from long-term inflammatory conditions.

3. Improves Immune Function

Ginger's ability to support the immune system makes it a popular remedy for fighting colds, flu, and infections. It is known for its antimicrobial and antiviral properties, which help the body combat harmful microorganisms. Ginger can stimulate the body's immune response, enhancing the activity of white blood cells that are responsible for fighting off infections.

Additionally, ginger's antioxidant properties help combat oxidative stress, which can weaken the immune system and increase susceptibility to infections. By neutralizing harmful free radicals, ginger helps maintain the health and function of the immune system, ensuring a stronger defense against viruses and bacteria.

4. Relieves Nausea and Morning Sickness

One of ginger's most well-known uses is its ability to relieve nausea. Whether you're dealing with motion sickness, morning sickness during pregnancy, or nausea caused by medical treatments such as chemotherapy, ginger has been shown to effectively alleviate symptoms.

In fact, multiple studies have confirmed ginger's ability to significantly reduce nausea in pregnant women. A typical dosage ranges from 500 mg to 1,000 mg of ginger powder per day, though it's best to consult with a healthcare provider before using ginger for morning sickness, especially during the early stages of pregnancy.

For those experiencing nausea related to chemotherapy, ginger can be particularly helpful. It is believed to reduce the frequency and severity of nausea episodes, improving the overall quality of life for cancer patients undergoing treatment.

5. Boosts Brain Function and Mental Clarity

Ginger has cognitive benefits that go beyond supporting general wellness. It contains bioactive compounds, like gingerol, that promote better brain function. Some studies suggest that ginger can improve memory, focus, and attention span, particularly in aging adults.

Ginger's neuroprotective effects are attributed to its potent antioxidant and anti-inflammatory properties. It helps protect brain cells from oxidative damage and inflammation, which are associated with cognitive decline and diseases like Alzheimer's and Parkinson's.

Regular consumption of ginger may help enhance mental clarity, focus, and memory, making it an ideal natural remedy for those seeking to improve mental sharpness, particularly for older individuals looking to protect against age-related cognitive decline.

6. Promotes Cardiovascular Health

Ginger has significant cardiovascular benefits, particularly in supporting heart health and circulation. It helps improve blood circulation and may reduce the risk of developing high blood pressure, heart disease, and stroke.

Ginger has been shown to lower cholesterol levels, particularly LDL (bad cholesterol), and increase HDL (good cholesterol). This contributes to improved circulation and a reduction in the buildup of fatty deposits in the arteries, which can contribute to atherosclerosis (hardening of the arteries).

Additionally, ginger has blood-thinning properties that can prevent blood clots from forming, thus reducing the risk of heart attack and stroke. It is often used as part of a heart-healthy diet to support overall cardiovascular function.

7. Supports Weight Management

Ginger can play a role in weight loss and weight management due to its ability to increase metabolism and reduce appetite. It has thermogenic properties, which means that it helps increase the body's heat production, leading to greater energy expenditure and fat burning.

Studies have shown that ginger can promote fat loss by stimulating lipolysis, the process by which fat cells break down and release stored fat. It may also help reduce food cravings and improve feelings of fullness after meals, which can prevent overeating.

Incorporating ginger into your diet as a part of a balanced weight loss plan can provide added support for fat burning and help you maintain a healthy weight.

8. Alleviates Menstrual Discomfort

Ginger has been used for centuries to alleviate the symptoms of menstrual cramps. It works by reducing the production of prostaglandins, which are hormone-like compounds responsible for causing the painful contractions of the uterus during menstruation.

Studies have shown that ginger is as effective as some over-the-counter pain medications, such as ibuprofen, in reducing menstrual pain. It can be consumed as a tea, capsule, or in powdered form to help alleviate the discomfort associated with menstrual cramps and to promote smoother menstrual cycles.

How to Incorporate Ginger into Your Routine

Ginger is a versatile root that can be used in a variety of ways to support your health and wellness. Here are some common methods of consuming ginger:

1. Fresh Ginger: The most potent form of ginger is fresh. It can be grated or sliced and added to a variety of dishes, from soups and stir-fries to smoothies and teas. Fresh ginger has a sharp, spicy flavor that adds depth to savory dishes and sweetness to drinks.

2. Ginger Tea: Ginger tea is one of the simplest and most popular ways to enjoy the health benefits of ginger. It can be made by boiling fresh ginger slices in water and adding lemon or honey for extra flavor. Ginger tea can be consumed throughout the day to help with digestion, nausea, and inflammation.

3. Ginger Capsules/Tablets: For those who prefer a more convenient option, ginger supplements are available in capsule or tablet form. Standard dosages range from 500 mg to 1,000 mg of ginger extract per day, typically divided into two or three doses.

4. Ginger Powder: Ginger powder is made by drying and grinding the root into a fine powder. It can be sprinkled into smoothies, shakes, or sprinkled over meals such as curries and stir-fries.

5. Ginger Extract/Tinctures: For those looking for a more concentrated dose, ginger extract or tinctures are available and can be added to water or other drinks.

These are potent options for those seeking quick relief from symptoms like nausea or joint pain.

6. Topical Application: Ginger can also be applied topically in the form of creams or oils to soothe muscle aches, joint pain, or inflammation. Ginger oil is often used in aromatherapy or massaged into the skin to promote relaxation and relieve tension.

Precautions and Side Effects

While ginger is generally safe for most people, it's important to be mindful of the following considerations:

1. Pregnancy: Pregnant women should consult with their healthcare provider before using ginger in large quantities, especially if they are using it for morning sickness. While ginger is generally considered safe in moderate amounts, excessive intake can lead to complications such as miscarriage or premature labor.

2. Blood Thinners: Ginger has natural blood-thinning properties and should be used cautiously by individuals taking blood-thinning medications like warfarin or aspirin. Excessive ginger consumption could increase the risk of bleeding.

3. Gastrointestinal Issues: While ginger can aid digestion, it can also cause heartburn, gas, or upset stomach in some individuals, particularly when consumed in large quantities. If you experience any

discomfort, it's best to reduce your intake and consult a healthcare provider if symptoms persist.

4. Allergies: Though rare, some individuals may have an allergic reaction to ginger. Signs of an allergy include skin rashes, itching, or swelling. If you suspect an allergy, discontinue use and seek medical advice.

5. Interaction with Medications: Ginger can interact with certain medications, including blood pressure medications, diabetes medications, and antacids. It's important to consult your healthcare provider before incorporating large amounts of ginger into your routine, especially if you are on prescribed medications.

6. Children: While ginger is safe for most children in small amounts, it's best to avoid giving large doses or supplements to young children without consulting a pediatrician, especially for medicinal purposes.

Embracing the Power of Ginger

Ginger is much more than just a flavorful addition to your meals—it's a versatile and powerful herb with a wide range of health benefits. From its ability to ease digestive discomfort and reduce inflammation to supporting cardiovascular health and enhancing cognitive function, ginger is an indispensable ally in promoting overall wellness.

Whether you choose to incorporate it into your diet through fresh ginger, tea, powder, or supplements, this root has stood the test of time as a natural remedy for various ailments. However, as with any natural treatment, it's important to use ginger responsibly and consult with a healthcare provider if you have underlying health conditions or concerns.

By adding ginger to your daily routine, you can harness its many health benefits and enjoy a healthier, more vibrant life. As always, remember that moderation is key, and a balanced approach to incorporating herbs and natural remedies into your wellness regimen will help you achieve optimal results.

Chapter 6: Neem – The Ancient Healer

For centuries, the neem tree (Azadirachta indica) has been revered in traditional medicine across India, Southeast Asia, and Africa. Known as the "village pharmacy" in India, neem has long been celebrated for its vast array of health benefits. With its roots deeply embedded in Ayurvedic and other holistic healing systems, neem's versatility and powerful medicinal properties make it one of the most potent plants in nature's pharmacy.

A Brief History of Neem

Neem is native to the Indian subcontinent but has since spread to tropical and subtropical regions of the world. The tree's use in traditional medicine dates back over 5,000 years, with every part of the neem tree – from its bark and leaves to its seeds and oil – being utilized for healing purposes. Ancient texts like the Charaka Samhita, one of the foundational texts of Ayurveda, mention neem as a powerful remedy for various ailments, ranging from skin disorders to digestive problems.

In modern times, neem's popularity has spread globally as researchers continue to uncover its incredible potential. From its antibacterial properties to its ability to support the immune system, neem has become a go-to remedy in holistic wellness practices. The tree's powerful properties lie within its unique chemical compounds, including azadirachtin, nimbin, and nimbolide, which contribute to its healing effects.

Neem's Powerful Medicinal Properties

Neem is often regarded as a "miracle herb" due to its broad-spectrum healing properties. Its many uses range from treating skin conditions and improving dental health to acting as an immune booster and a powerful detoxifier.

1. Antibacterial, Antifungal, and Antiviral Properties: One of neem's most notable benefits is its strong antibacterial, antifungal, and antiviral capabilities. Neem has been used to treat a wide range of infections, including skin infections like eczema, acne, and fungal infections like athlete's foot. Its ability to combat harmful bacteria and fungi makes it an excellent natural alternative to chemical-based treatments. It's also used to treat viral infections like chickenpox, herpes, and warts, showing its versatility as a broad-spectrum antimicrobial agent.

2. Immune System Support: Neem has powerful immunomodulatory effects, meaning it can both boost and regulate the immune system. For individuals suffering from autoimmune conditions or compromised immunity, neem helps balance immune responses, reducing inflammation and strengthening the body's defenses against infections. By promoting

the production of white blood cells, neem aids in fighting off harmful pathogens while reducing the body's susceptibility to illness.

3. Detoxification: Neem plays an essential role in detoxifying the body. It supports the liver by helping to neutralize and remove toxins, improving overall liver function. This detoxifying effect extends to the blood as well, as neem helps purify the blood by removing impurities and boosting circulation. Regular use of neem can promote clearer skin and reduce the occurrence of skin blemishes and rashes caused by internal toxins.

4. Anti-inflammatory Effects: Chronic inflammation is at the root of many modern health conditions, including arthritis, heart disease, and autoimmune disorders. Neem's potent anti-inflammatory properties can help reduce inflammation and alleviate symptoms associated with conditions like rheumatoid arthritis and osteoarthritis. Its compounds inhibit the production of pro-inflammatory molecules, helping to soothe inflammation both internally and externally.

Neem and Skin Health

One of neem's most popular uses today is for skincare. The leaves and oil of the neem tree are widely used in natural skincare products due to their ability to treat acne, blemishes, and other skin conditions. Neem's antibacterial properties help cleanse the skin, making it an effective treatment for acne and pimples. It also has anti-inflammatory effects, which help reduce the redness and swelling that often accompany skin breakouts.

Neem oil is known for its ability to fight fungal infections such as athlete's foot, ringworm, and dandruff. Its antifungal and antimicrobial properties work to cleanse the scalp, reduce irritation, and restore balance to the skin.

Additionally, neem's ability to promote cell regeneration makes it a fantastic remedy for aging skin. It can help reduce the appearance of wrinkles and fine lines while promoting the healing of scars and sun damage. Regular use of neem-based products can improve overall skin texture, leaving it feeling soft, smooth, and rejuvenated.

Oral Health: Neem's Role in Dental Care

In many parts of the world, neem has been used for centuries to maintain oral hygiene. The practice of chewing on neem twigs, known as "datun" in India, is still common in rural areas due to its antibacterial and antiseptic properties. Neem's ability to fight bacteria and germs makes it an effective natural remedy for maintaining healthy teeth and gums.

Neem can help fight the bacteria that cause gum disease, cavities, and bad breath. Its antimicrobial properties also promote overall oral hygiene by reducing plaque buildup, preventing gingivitis, and soothing irritated gums. Neem-based toothpaste and mouthwashes are widely available, providing a natural alternative to chemical-laden oral care products.

How to Incorporate Neem Into Your Life

Neem can be incorporated into your daily routine in several ways, whether in the form of oil, capsules, powder, or tea. Here are some practical ways to incorporate neem into your health regimen:

Neem Oil: Neem oil is highly concentrated and can be used topically to treat skin conditions, such as acne, eczema, psoriasis, and fungal infections. It can also be applied to the scalp to combat dandruff and promote healthy hair growth. Due to its potency, neem oil should be diluted with a carrier oil (such as coconut or olive oil) before applying it to the skin.

Neem Powder: Neem powder is available as a supplement or in loose powder form. You can mix the powder with water, juice, or smoothies. For those interested in detoxification or immune support, neem powder can be taken in capsule form for convenience.

Neem Tea: Drinking neem tea can support the body's detoxification process and improve skin health. Simply steep fresh neem leaves or neem powder in hot water for a few minutes and enjoy this cleansing, immune-boosting beverage. Neem tea can also help regulate blood sugar levels and improve digestive health.

Neem-Based Products: For skincare, neem is commonly found in soaps, lotions, and creams. These products are designed to soothe and heal the skin while fighting bacteria and promoting cell regeneration.

Is Neem Right for You?

While neem is generally safe for most people, there are a few considerations to keep in mind. Neem is known to lower blood sugar levels, so people with diabetes or those taking medications for blood sugar regulation should consult with their healthcare provider before using neem products. Pregnant and breastfeeding women should also exercise caution, as neem can have a strong effect on the body and may not be suitable during these periods.

It's always recommended to perform a patch test when using neem oil or topical products to ensure that you don't have an allergic reaction. If irritation occurs, discontinue use immediately.

Final Thoughts on Neem

Neem is a powerhouse herb with an impressive range of health benefits. Its antibacterial, antifungal, antiviral, and anti-inflammatory properties make it a versatile and valuable addition to any wellness routine. Whether you're using it to improve your skin health, boost your immune system, or detoxify your body, neem offers a natural and effective solution to many modern health challenges.

By incorporating neem into your daily life, you can tap into the ancient wisdom of this remarkable plant and experience its numerous healing benefits. As with any herb or supplement, it's important to consult with a healthcare provider before beginning any new regimen, especially if you have pre-existing health conditions or are taking medication.

Chapter 8: Baobab – The Tree of Life

In the heart of Africa's vast landscapes stands a tree of mythical proportions, a life-giving marvel revered for its resilience and abundance. The baobab tree, often called "The Tree of Life," is not just a botanical wonder; it is a symbol of nourishment, sustainability, and survival for communities living in some of the harshest climates on Earth. Every part of this ancient tree—its leaves, bark, seeds, and fruit—offers remarkable health benefits, earning it a place of honor in traditional medicine and modern nutrition.

This chapter explores the baobab tree's history, its nutritional profile, and its profound impact on health and wellness.

The Legacy of the Baobab Tree

The baobab tree *Adansonia digitata* is one of nature's oldest living organisms, with some trees believed to be over 2,000 years old. Native to Africa, baobabs are also found in Madagascar, Australia, and the Arabian Peninsula. The tree's unique, bulbous trunk can store thousands of liters of water, enabling it to survive in arid climates and provide sustenance during droughts.

In African folklore, the baobab is known as the "upside-down tree" because of its bare, root-like branches. It is central to many myths and cultural practices, symbolizing wisdom, strength, and longevity.

Traditionally, the baobab tree has been a communal meeting point, a place for storytelling, ceremonies, and even refuge.

Nutritional Powerhouse: The Baobab Fruit

The baobab fruit, often referred to as "superfruit," is the most celebrated part of the tree. Encased in a hard shell, the fruit pulp is naturally dehydrated, making it easy to store and use. Its nutritional profile is unparalleled:

Vitamin C: Baobab fruit contains up to 10 times more vitamin C than oranges, making it a powerful immune booster.

Antioxidants: Rich in polyphenols, baobab offers one of the highest antioxidant contents among fruits, helping combat oxidative stress and inflammation.

Fiber: The fruit pulp is nearly 50% fiber, which supports digestion and gut health.

Minerals: Baobab is a great source of calcium, magnesium, potassium, and iron, essential for bone health, muscle function, and energy production.

The fruit also contains a low glycemic index, making it an ideal addition to diets focused on blood sugar control.

Health Benefits of Baobab

1. Immune System Support

Baobab's high vitamin C content makes it a natural ally in strengthening the immune system. Vitamin C stimulates the production of white blood cells, enhances wound healing, and acts as a powerful antioxidant to protect the body from free radical damage.

2. Digestive Health

The soluble and insoluble fiber in baobab supports digestive health by promoting regular bowel movements and feeding beneficial gut bacteria. This prebiotic effect helps maintain a healthy microbiome, which is crucial for overall health.

Studies have shown that baobab fiber can also aid in reducing inflammation in the gut, making it beneficial for people with conditions like irritable bowel syndrome (IBS) and inflammatory bowel disease (IBD).

3. Blood Sugar Regulation

Baobab's fiber slows down the absorption of sugars into the bloodstream, preventing spikes in blood sugar levels. This makes it particularly helpful for people with diabetes or those at risk of developing the condition.

A study published in Nutrition Research found that consuming baobab fruit extract reduced the glycemic response to carbohydrate-rich meals, making it a natural option for managing blood sugar levels.

4. Skin Health

The antioxidants and vitamin C in baobab promote collagen production, essential for maintaining the skin's elasticity and youthful appearance. Baobab oil, extracted from the seeds, is widely used in skincare products to hydrate and nourish the skin. It is especially effective for treating dry skin, scars, and stretch marks.

5. Energy and Hydration

Baobab is a natural energy booster due to its rich combination of vitamins, minerals, and antioxidants. Its potassium content helps replenish electrolytes, making it an excellent choice for athletes or those recovering from dehydration.

6. Bone and Joint Health

Baobab is a significant source of calcium and magnesium, minerals essential for maintaining strong bones and preventing osteoporosis. Its anti-inflammatory properties also help alleviate joint pain and stiffness, making it a valuable addition to diets for individuals with arthritis.

7. Weight Management

Baobab's high fiber content promotes satiety, reducing overall calorie intake. Incorporating baobab into meals can help control hunger and support weight loss efforts.

Traditional Uses of Baobab

Baobab has been used in traditional medicine for centuries. Here are some examples of how different parts of the tree have been utilized:

Leaves: The young leaves are rich in calcium, iron, and protein. They are often dried and powdered to make a nutritious supplement for children and pregnant women. They are also used to treat fevers, diarrhea, and respiratory issues.

Bark: The bark is used to make ropes and fabrics, but it also has medicinal applications. It is boiled to create a remedy for fevers, malaria, and infections.

Seeds: The seeds are roasted and consumed as snacks or pressed to extract oil. Baobab seed oil is highly valued for its emollient properties in skincare.

Fruit Pulp: The fruit pulp is dissolved in water to create a refreshing drink, often used to treat dehydration and heat exhaustion.

Incorporating Baobab into Your Diet

Baobab fruit powder is now widely available and can be easily incorporated into your daily routine. Here are some ideas:

Smoothies: Add a tablespoon of baobab powder to your favorite smoothie for a tangy, citrusy flavor and a nutrient boost.

Baking: Mix baobab powder into muffins, cookies, or pancakes for added fiber and vitamins.

Drinks: Stir baobab powder into water or juice for a quick and refreshing drink.

Yogurt and Oatmeal: Sprinkle baobab powder over yogurt or oatmeal for a nutritious topping.

Sustainability and Ethical Harvesting

Baobab trees play a critical role in the ecosystems where they grow. They provide food and shelter for animals and support local communities by offering a sustainable source of income. Ethical harvesting of baobab fruit ensures that the trees are not damaged and can continue to thrive for future generations.

By choosing baobab products from reputable sources, you can support conservation efforts and fair trade practices, ensuring that the benefits of this incredible tree are shared equitably.

Precautions and Considerations

While baobab is generally safe for most people, some individuals may experience allergic reactions or digestive discomfort. It is advisable to start with small amounts if you are new to baobab and consult a healthcare provider if you have any underlying health conditions or concerns.

The baobab tree is a testament to nature's generosity, offering nourishment, health, and sustainability in every part of its being. From its nutrient-dense fruit to its medicinal leaves and bark, baobab has earned its title as the "Tree of Life."

By incorporating baobab into your diet and lifestyle, you can tap into the wealth of health benefits this ancient tree provides while supporting ethical and sustainable practices. In a world searching for natural, effective health solutions, baobab stands as a shining example of the healing power of nature.

Chapter 9: Amaranth – The Ancient Grain of Vitality

Amaranth, a grain revered by ancient civilizations, continues to hold a prominent place in the world of nutrition. Once considered a sacred crop by the Aztecs and Incas, amaranth has gained recognition worldwide as a superfood, prized for its versatility, resilience, and impressive nutrient profile. This chapter delves into the history, nutritional significance, and health benefits of amaranth, highlighting why it deserves a spot in your pantry.

A Brief History of Amaranth

Amaranth, belonging to the genus Amaranthus, is not technically a grain but a "pseudo-cereal" like quinoa and buckwheat. Indigenous to Central and South America, it was a staple in the diets of the Aztecs, who called it huāuhtli. It was used not only as food but also in religious rituals, symbolizing life and fertility.

When Spanish conquistadors arrived, they sought to suppress its cultivation due to its cultural and religious significance. Despite this, amaranth survived in remote areas and was later reintroduced to the world as a resilient and nutritious crop.

Today, amaranth is grown globally, from Africa to Asia, for its leaves, seeds, and ability to thrive in harsh conditions.

The Nutritional Powerhouse

Amaranth is packed with essential nutrients, offering a comprehensive blend of macronutrients and micronutrients. Here's what makes it stand out:

Protein: Amaranth is one of the few plant-based sources of complete protein, containing all nine essential amino acids. This makes it particularly valuable for vegetarians and vegans.

Fiber: High in dietary fiber, amaranth supports digestion and promotes satiety.

Minerals: It is rich in calcium, magnesium, iron, and phosphorus, which are essential for bone health, energy production, and red blood cell formation.

Vitamins: Amaranth contains B vitamins, including folate, which are vital for energy metabolism and DNA synthesis.

Antioxidants: Amaranth is loaded with antioxidants, such as phenolic compounds, which protect cells from damage caused by free radicals.

Gluten-Free: As a naturally gluten-free grain, amaranth is an excellent choice for people with celiac disease or gluten intolerance.

Health Benefits of Amaranth

1. Boosts Protein Intake

Amaranth's high protein content is its most celebrated feature. With about 9 grams of protein per cooked cup, it supports muscle repair, tissue growth, and overall bodily function. Its amino acid profile, especially lysine, sets it apart from other grains, as lysine is often lacking in plant-based diets.

2. Promotes Digestive Health

The fiber in amaranth aids in maintaining regular bowel movements and preventing constipation. Additionally, fiber feeds the good bacteria in the gut, supporting a healthy microbiome and improving overall digestive health.

3. Supports Bone Health

Rich in calcium and magnesium, amaranth strengthens bones and teeth, making it an excellent addition for individuals at risk of osteoporosis. One cup of cooked amaranth provides about 12% of the daily calcium requirement.

4. Enhances Heart Health

Amaranth contains phytosterols and squalene, compounds known to reduce cholesterol levels. Its magnesium content helps relax blood vessels, lowering blood pressure and improving overall cardiovascular health.

5. Aids in Anemia Prevention

Iron-rich amaranth supports the production of hemoglobin and red blood cells, reducing the risk of iron-deficiency anemia. Combining amaranth with vitamin C-rich foods enhances iron absorption.

6. Manages Blood Sugar Levels

Amaranth's complex carbohydrates and fiber slow the digestion and absorption of sugars, preventing blood sugar spikes. This makes it a suitable food for individuals managing diabetes.

7. Antioxidant and Anti-Inflammatory Effects

The antioxidants in amaranth reduce oxidative stress and inflammation, lowering the risk of chronic diseases such as cancer, diabetes, and arthritis.

8. Weight Management

Amaranth's high fiber and protein content promote feelings of fullness, helping control appetite and reducing overall calorie intake.

Traditional and Culinary Uses

Amaranth is a versatile crop, with every part of the plant offering culinary or medicinal value.

Seeds: Used as a grain, the seeds can be cooked like rice, popped like popcorn, or ground into flour for baking.

Leaves: Amaranth leaves are rich in iron, calcium, and vitamins A and C. They are used in soups, stews, or as a leafy green in salads.

Stalks: The tender stalks are cooked and consumed in various traditional dishes.

Some common ways to incorporate amaranth into meals include:

Breakfast Porridge: Cook amaranth seeds with milk or water, adding fruits and nuts for a nutrient-rich start to the day.

Salads: Use cooked amaranth as a base for grain salads, mixing it with vegetables, herbs, and a tangy dressing.

Soups and Stews: Add amaranth seeds to soups for added texture and nutrition.

Baking: Amaranth flour can replace a portion of wheat flour in recipes for bread, pancakes, or muffins.

Popped Amaranth: Lightly heat the seeds in a dry skillet to create a crunchy, nutty snack or cereal topping.

Amaranth in Traditional Medicine

Amaranth has been used in traditional medicine for various purposes:

Wound Healing: Amaranth leaves were crushed and applied to wounds to promote healing.

Digestive Aid: A decoction of amaranth seeds or leaves was used to treat diarrhea and stomach discomfort.

Anti-Inflammatory: The leaves and seeds were used to reduce inflammation and fever.

Skin Health: Amaranth extracts were applied to the skin to alleviate rashes and dryness.

Sustainability and Global Importance

Amaranth is a drought-resistant crop, making it a lifeline in arid regions. It grows quickly, requires minimal water, and thrives in poor soil, providing food security for vulnerable populations. Organizations like the Food and Agriculture Organization (FAO) have promoted amaranth cultivation as a sustainable solution to global hunger and malnutrition.

Its role in crop rotation also improves soil health, as it prevents erosion and enhances soil fertility.

Precautions and Considerations

While amaranth is generally safe, some individuals may need to exercise caution:

Oxalates: Amaranth contains oxalates, which can contribute to kidney stones in susceptible individuals. Cooking and consuming amaranth in moderation can minimize this risk.

Allergies: Though rare, some people may have allergies to amaranth. Start with small quantities if you're trying it for the first time.

Amaranth's rich history, robust nutritional profile, and numerous health benefits make it a standout superfood. From ancient rituals to modern plates, it has proven to be a versatile, sustainable, and health-promoting crop.

By incorporating amaranth into your diet, you not only enhance your health but also support sustainable agricultural practices. In a world seeking resilient and nutritious food sources, amaranth truly embodies the spirit of vitality and abundance.

Chapter 10: Aloe Vera – The Plant of Immortality

Aloe vera, often called the "plant of immortality," has been treasured for its healing properties for thousands of years. With its fleshy, spiky leaves and cooling gel, this hardy succulent is a cornerstone of natural medicine, skincare, and wellness practices across the globe. In this chapter, we explore the origins, science-backed benefits, and versatile uses of aloe vera, a plant that has stood the test of time.

A Glimpse Into History

Aloe vera's use dates back over 6,000 years to ancient Egypt, where it was revered as a symbol of immortality. Cleopatra and Nefertiti are said to have used aloe gel in their beauty routines. The ancient Greeks, Chinese, and Indians also embraced aloe vera for its medicinal and cosmetic properties.

Aloe vera later spread across the globe, carried by traders and explorers. Its ability to thrive in arid climates made it a staple in regions ranging from the Arabian Peninsula to Central America.

The Anatomy of Aloe Vera

The aloe vera plant *Aloe barbadensis miller* is prized for the gel and latex it produces:

Aloe Gel: The clear, viscous substance inside the leaves contains over 75 active compounds, including vitamins, enzymes, amino acids, and polysaccharides.

Aloe Latex: The yellowish sap beneath the leaf's skin contains aloin, a compound with laxative properties.

These components work synergistically to provide aloe vera's wide-ranging health benefits.

Nutritional and Medicinal Components

Aloe vera is a powerhouse of bioactive compounds:

Vitamins: Rich in vitamins A, C, and E, aloe vera provides antioxidant protection. It also contains vitamin B12, crucial for nerve health.

Minerals: Contains calcium, magnesium, zinc, and potassium, essential for various bodily functions.

Enzymes: Includes amylase and lipase, which aid in digestion, and bradykinase, known for reducing inflammation.

Polysaccharides: These sugars enhance skin hydration, support wound healing, and boost immunity.

Amino Acids: Aloe vera contains 20 of the 22 essential amino acids the body requires for protein synthesis.

Plant Sterols: Known for their anti-inflammatory and cholesterol-lowering effects.

Health Benefits of Aloe Vera

1. Soothes Skin Irritations

Aloe vera is perhaps best known for its ability to treat skin conditions. Its gel provides instant relief for burns, sunburns, cuts, and insect bites. It accelerates wound healing by increasing collagen production and improving blood flow to the affected area.

2. Hydrates and Nourishes the Skin

Aloe gel is a natural humectant, drawing moisture into the skin. It reduces dryness and promotes a youthful glow. Regular use can help manage acne, eczema, and psoriasis.

3. Supports Digestive Health

Aloe vera juice has been traditionally used to soothe the digestive tract. It aids in managing conditions like acid reflux, irritable bowel syndrome (IBS), and constipation, thanks to its anti-inflammatory and laxative properties.

4. Strengthens the Immune System

The polysaccharides in aloe vera boost the immune response by stimulating white blood cell production. This enhances the body's ability to fight off infections and illnesses.

5. Reduces Inflammation

Aloe vera contains compounds like bradykinase and salicylic acid, which help reduce inflammation in the skin, joints, and internal organs.

6. Promotes Oral Health

Aloe vera is effective in treating gum diseases like gingivitis and periodontitis. Its antimicrobial properties reduce plaque buildup and soothe swollen gums.

7. Regulates Blood Sugar

Emerging research suggests that aloe vera may help lower blood glucose levels, making it a potential aid for people with type 2 diabetes.

8. Enhances Hair Health

Aloe vera gel nourishes the scalp, reduces dandruff, and strengthens hair follicles. Its enzymes promote healthy hair growth by removing dead skin cells that clog pores.

Traditional and Modern Uses

Aloe vera's versatility extends beyond health remedies:

Skincare Products: Found in moisturizers, sunscreens, and anti-aging creams, aloe vera soothes and protects the skin.

Beverages: Aloe vera juice is consumed for its digestive and detoxifying properties.

Hair Care: Shampoos and conditioners infused with aloe vera improve hair texture and scalp health.

Wound Healing: Aloe vera gel is applied to minor cuts, scrapes, and burns for faster recovery.

Household Remedies: A diluted aloe solution can be used as a natural disinfectant for minor surfaces.

How to Use Aloe Vera

For Skincare

1. Cut an aloe vera leaf and scoop out the gel.

2. Apply the gel directly to your skin for hydration or to treat sunburn, acne, or eczema.

3. Mix it with coconut oil or honey for a DIY face mask.

For Hair Care

1. Massage fresh aloe gel into your scalp and hair.

2. Leave it on for 20-30 minutes before rinsing for softer, shinier hair.

For Digestive Health

1. Drink a small amount of aloe vera juice (about 30-50 ml) to soothe the digestive tract.

2. Avoid consuming too much, as it may have a laxative effect.

Sustainability and Cultivation

Aloe vera is a low-maintenance plant that thrives in arid climates. It requires minimal water and is resistant to pests, making it an environmentally friendly crop. Its rapid growth rate and medicinal properties have led to its widespread cultivation in home gardens and commercial farms alike.

Precautions and Side Effects

While aloe vera is generally safe, it's important to use it responsibly:

Topical Use: Rarely, aloe vera may cause allergic reactions. Always perform a patch test before applying it to your skin.

Oral Consumption: Excessive consumption of aloe latex can cause cramping, diarrhea, and dehydration. Pregnant and breastfeeding women should avoid it.

Medication Interactions: Aloe vera may interact with certain medications, such as diabetes drugs and diuretics. Consult a healthcare professional before use.

Aloe vera is a timeless remedy that bridges the gap between ancient wisdom and modern science. Whether soothing a burn, hydrating your skin, or supporting your digestive health, this "plant of immortality" continues to prove its worth.

By incorporating aloe vera into your routine, you tap into a natural source of healing and vitality that has stood the test of time. Accessible, versatile, and sustainable, aloe vera is a true gift from nature, offering benefits for both your health and beauty.

Chapter 11: Hibiscus – The Heart-Friendly Flower

Hibiscus, with its striking red petals and tart, refreshing flavor, has earned a place as one of the most cherished medicinal plants in the world. Known for its vibrant beauty and therapeutic properties, this flowering plant is revered for its role in promoting heart health and overall wellness. In this chapter, we explore the origins, health benefits, and ways to incorporate hibiscus into your daily life.

A Journey Through History

The use of hibiscus dates back thousands of years, with its roots in ancient Egypt. Pharaohs drank hibiscus tea, known as karkadeh, to cool their bodies in the desert heat. In Ayurveda and traditional Chinese medicine, hibiscus has been used for its cooling, diuretic, and heart-supporting properties.

Hibiscus soon traveled across the globe, becoming a staple in African, Caribbean, and Latin American cultures. Today, it remains a key ingredient in herbal medicine and culinary traditions worldwide.

The Anatomy of Hibiscus

The most commonly used species for medicinal purposes is Hibiscus sabdariffa, also known as roselle. The plant's calyces—the cup-like structures at the base of the flower—are rich in beneficial compounds, including:

Antioxidants: Polyphenols and anthocyanins that combat oxidative stress.

Vitamins: High levels of Vitamin C and A, which support immunity and skin health.

Minerals: Iron, magnesium, and potassium, essential for heart and muscle function.

Acids: Organic acids like citric and malic acid, which give hibiscus its tangy taste and detoxifying properties.

Health Benefits of Hibiscus

1. Supports Heart Health

Hibiscus is most famous for its ability to lower blood pressure. Studies show that drinking hibiscus tea regularly can significantly reduce both systolic and diastolic blood pressure, making it a natural alternative for hypertension management. Its diuretic properties help the body eliminate excess sodium, further aiding heart health.

2. Lowers Cholesterol Levels

Hibiscus contains compounds that help reduce LDL (bad cholesterol) levels and increase HDL (good cholesterol). This dual action protects against heart disease and supports cardiovascular health.

3. Regulates Blood Sugar

Research suggests that hibiscus tea may help stabilize blood sugar levels, making it beneficial for people with diabetes or those at risk of developing the condition.

4. Boosts Immunity

Rich in Vitamin C and powerful antioxidants, hibiscus strengthens the immune system, helping the body fight off infections and reduce inflammation.

5. Aids Digestion

Hibiscus has mild laxative properties, which can help relieve constipation and promote a healthy digestive system. Its anti-inflammatory compounds also soothe the gastrointestinal tract.

6. Promotes Weight Management

Hibiscus tea may inhibit the production of amylase, an enzyme that breaks down starches into sugars. This action helps slow carbohydrate absorption and supports weight management efforts.

7. Protects the Liver

Antioxidants in hibiscus protect the liver from damage caused by toxins and free radicals. Regular consumption can improve liver function and promote detoxification.

8. Enhances Skin Health

The high antioxidant content of hibiscus helps combat signs of aging, such as wrinkles and fine lines. Its natural acids gently exfoliate the skin, leaving it smooth and glowing.

How to Use Hibiscus

Hibiscus Tea

1. Boil 1-2 tablespoons of dried hibiscus calyces in 2 cups of water for 5-10 minutes.

2. Strain and sweeten with honey or stevia, if desired.

3. Enjoy it hot or chilled as a refreshing beverage.

Hibiscus Syrup

1. Simmer hibiscus petals with sugar and water until it reduces into a thick syrup.

2. Use it to flavor cocktails, desserts, or pancakes.

Hibiscus Hair Rinse

1. Steep dried hibiscus in hot water, let it cool, and use it as a natural hair rinse.

2. This helps strengthen the hair, reduce dandruff, and enhance shine.

Hibiscus Face Mask

1. Blend dried hibiscus petals into a fine powder and mix with yogurt or honey.

2. Apply to the face for 10-15 minutes to rejuvenate and hydrate the skin.

Cultural and Culinary Significance

Hibiscus plays a vital role in the culinary traditions of many cultures:

Africa: In West Africa, hibiscus is used to make bissap, a popular drink served at celebrations.

Caribbean: Hibiscus tea is a holiday staple, often spiced with ginger and cloves.

Mexico: Known as agua de Jamaica, hibiscus tea is enjoyed as a sweet-tart beverage.

Thailand: Hibiscus flowers are candied and used as garnishes for desserts.

Precautions and Side Effects

While hibiscus is generally safe, it's important to be aware of potential side effects:

Blood Pressure: Individuals with low blood pressure should consume hibiscus in moderation, as it may further lower blood pressure.

Pregnancy and Breastfeeding: Pregnant and breastfeeding women should avoid hibiscus due to its potential to stimulate uterine contractions.

Medication Interactions: Hibiscus may interact with diuretics and medications for high blood pressure or diabetes.

Always consult a healthcare provider before incorporating hibiscus into your regimen, especially if you are on medication or have a medical condition.

Growing Hibiscus at Home

Hibiscus thrives in tropical and subtropical climates but can also be grown in pots indoors in cooler regions. Here are a few tips:

1. Planting: Choose a sunny location with well-drained soil.

2. Watering: Water regularly but avoid overwatering, as hibiscus is prone to root rot.

3. Pruning: Trim the plant to encourage bushier growth and more blooms.

4. Harvesting: Pick the calyces once the flowers have withered for optimal potency.

Hibiscus is a true gift from nature, offering vibrant beauty and a host of health benefits. Its ability to support heart health, regulate blood sugar, and enhance skin makes it an invaluable addition to your wellness routine.

Whether enjoyed as a soothing tea, a refreshing syrup, or a natural beauty remedy, hibiscus connects us to ancient traditions while meeting the demands of modern life. By embracing hibiscus, you're not just nurturing your body—you're celebrating a plant that has sustained cultures and generations across the globe.

Chapter 12: How to Incorporate These Plants into Your Life

Now that we've explored the incredible health benefits of nature's most powerful plants, the next step is making them a part of your daily routine. This chapter is your ultimate guide to seamlessly integrating these superfoods into your diet and lifestyle, ensuring you maximize their benefits without complicating your day.

Whether you're new to plant-based wellness or looking for fresh ideas, this chapter offers practical tips, recipes, and strategies to incorporate these plants into meals, beverages, and self-care routines.

Start Simple: One Plant at a Time

It's tempting to jump in and try everything at once, but introducing one plant at a time allows you to understand its effects on your body. For example, start with moringa for energy, then add spirulina or turmeric as you get comfortable.

Tip: Keep a journal to track how each plant makes you feel—energy levels, digestion, or overall wellness.

Morning Rituals: Energize Your Day

Smoothies: Start your day with a nutrient-packed smoothie. Combine fruits, a base (like almond milk or water), and a teaspoon of spirulina, chlorella, or baobab powder for an energy boost.

Herbal Teas: Brew hibiscus tea to jumpstart your metabolism or enjoy turmeric tea with ginger and honey for an anti-inflammatory kick.

Supplements: Capsules of ashwagandha, neem, or gotu kola can easily fit into your morning vitamin routine.

Recipe Idea:

Green Energy Smoothie

- ✓ 1 banana
- ✓ 1 cup spinach
- ✓ 1/2 cup frozen pineapple
- ✓ 1 tsp moringa powder
- ✓ 1 cup coconut water

Blend until smooth and enjoy a refreshing burst of nutrients!

Midday Boost: Healthy Snacks and Lunch Ideas

Incorporating plants into your midday meals is easier than you think:

Salads: Sprinkle toasted amaranth seeds or chopped purslane over your salad for added crunch and nutrition.

Soups: Add a spoonful of wheatgrass powder to vegetable soup or stew for a subtle, earthy flavor.

Snack Bars: Mix baobab powder into homemade granola bars for a tangy Vitamin C boost.

Recipe Idea:

Baobab Superfood Salad

- ✓ 2 cups mixed greens
- ✓ 1/4 cup pomegranate seeds
- ✓ 1 tbsp baobab powder (whisked into the dressing)
- ✓ 2 tbsp olive oil, 1 tbsp lemon juice, salt, and pepper for the dressing.

Evening Wind-Down: Relax and Restore

Golden Milk: Enjoy a warm mug of golden milk before bed. Mix turmeric, ashwagandha powder, and a dash of cinnamon into warm almond milk for a soothing anti-inflammatory drink.

Calming Teas: Brew gotu kola tea to unwind and support brain health after a long day.

Face Masks: Create a DIY aloe vera or hibiscus face mask to pamper your skin while you relax.

Recipe Idea:

Golden Turmeric Milk

- ✓ 1 cup almond milk
- ✓ 1/2 tsp turmeric
- ✓ 1/4 tsp cinnamon
- ✓ 1/4 tsp ashwagandha powder
- ✓ Sweetener of choice (honey or stevia)

Heat and whisk until smooth.

Recipes for the Entire Family

Incorporating these plants isn't just for adults—they're great for kids too!

Popsicles: Blend hibiscus tea, honey, and fresh berries, then freeze for a refreshing treat.

Baked Goods: Add amaranth flour to muffins or pancakes for a nutrient-rich twist.

Sprinkled Powders: Sprinkle baobab or wheatgrass powder into your child's yogurt or cereal.

Creative Ways to Use These Plants

1. Cooking with Superfoods

Turmeric: Add to curries, roasted vegetables, or rice dishes.

Neem: Incorporate neem powder into smoothies or teas for a detoxifying boost.

Amaranth: Use as a base for porridge or as a replacement for rice.

2. DIY Beauty Products

Aloe Vera: Use fresh aloe gel as a moisturizer or mix with essential oils for a hair mask.

Hibiscus: Make a hydrating toner by steeping hibiscus in water and storing it in a spray bottle.

3. Home Remedies

Wheatgrass Juice: Drink fresh wheatgrass shots for an immunity boost.

Neem Oil: Use neem oil as a natural insect repellent or to soothe irritated skin.

On-the-Go Solutions

For busy lifestyles, convenience is key:

Pre-Mixed Powders: Purchase high-quality blends of spirulina, chlorella, or wheatgrass to add to water or juice.

Snack Packs: Carry energy bars made with baobab, moringa, or amaranth for a quick, healthy snack.

Tea Bags: Keep hibiscus or ashwagandha tea bags in your bag for instant relaxation.

Sourcing and Storing Superfoods

Where to Find Them

Local Markets: Check health food stores or farmer's markets for fresh and dried options.

Online Retailers: Look for certified organic and non-GMO products.

Grow Your Own: Plants like wheatgrass, aloe vera, and purslane are easy to cultivate at home.

How to Store Them

Powders: Store in airtight containers in a cool, dry place.

Fresh Leaves: Keep in the refrigerator and use within a week.

Oils: Store in dark bottles to prevent oxidation.

A Final Word: Making It a Lifestyle

Incorporating these plants into your life isn't about perfection—it's about making small, sustainable changes that benefit your health over time. Start by experimenting with one or two plants, find what works best for your needs, and gradually expand your repertoire.

By embracing these superfoods, you're not just nourishing your body—you're connecting with centuries of traditional wisdom and the healing power of nature.

So, let your journey with these plants begin. From teas to tinctures, smoothies to salads, there are endless ways to enjoy the benefits of these green elixirs. Here's to a healthier, more vibrant you!

Embracing Nature's Green Elixirs

Nature has always held the key to wellness. Through the leaves, roots, flowers, and fruits of its incredible bounty, it provides remedies and nutrients that modern science is only beginning to fully understand. As we've journeyed through the remarkable properties of plants like moringa, spirulina, turmeric, baobab, aloe vera, and many others, one thing is clear: the path to health is often as simple as returning to nature.

By incorporating these plants into your daily life, you're not just consuming food—you're embracing a philosophy. A philosophy that values balance, holistic wellness, and respect for the environment. These green elixirs remind us that health doesn't come in a single pill but in the vibrant variety of nature's offerings.

As you take your first steps into the world of plant-based healing, remember:

Start small and stay consistent.

Experiment with flavors, forms, and recipes until you find what resonates with you.

And above all, listen to your body—it is the best guide to what works for you.

The plants discussed in this book are more than nutritional powerhouses; they are bridges to a healthier, more harmonious life. By adopting even a few of these plants into your routine, you can unlock their immense potential, transforming not just your physical health but your overall well-being.

Let this book serve as a foundation and a source of inspiration. Continue exploring, learning, and experimenting with nature's gifts. Together, we can move toward a world that appreciates and thrives on the sustainable power of plants.

Here's to your journey of vibrant health and the timeless healing wisdom of nature.

About the Author

Caterinah Muiruri is a passionate enthusiast of natural health and wellness with a deep curiosity about the healing power of plants. Though not a professional in the field, their journey into plant-based living began with a personal quest for better health and a desire to reconnect with nature.

Driven by a love for learning and a commitment to holistic well-being, Caterinah has spent countless hours researching the nutritional and medicinal properties of plants. They believe that the wisdom of nature is accessible to everyone, and their goal is to inspire others to explore the benefits of these incredible natural resources.

With a knack for simplifying complex information and making it approachable, Caterinah hopes to empower readers to make informed choices about their health. They see themselves not as an expert, but as a fellow traveler on the path to natural wellness, eager to share what they've discovered along the way.

When not writing or experimenting with plant-based remedies, Caterinah cooking, drawing, traveling, spending time in nature, trying new recipes, or exploring local markets for fresh ingredients.

The Green Elixir: Unlocking the Health Benefits of Nature's Most Powerful Plants is a reflection of their passion for plant-based healing and their desire to inspire others to embrace the power of nature in their everyday lives.

9 798305 497786